T0320967

KNOWLEDGE INTO ACTION

A GUIDE TO RESEARCH UTILIZATION

GEORGE P. CERNADA

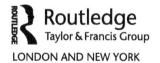

Routledge
Taylor & Francis Group

LONDON AND NEW YORK

First published 1982 by Baywood Publishing Company, Inc.

2 Park Square, Milton Park, Abingdon, Oxfordshire OX14 4RN
52 Vanderbilt Avenue, New York, NY 10017

Routledge is an imprint of the Taylor & Francis Group, an informa business

First issued in hardback 2019

Library of Congress Catalog Card Number 81-20482

Library of Congress Cataloging in Publication Data
    Main entry under title:
Cernada, George P. (George Peter)
    Knowledge into Action.
    Includes bibliographical references.
    1. Sociology — Research — Case studies. 2. Underdeveloped areas — Community health services — Case studies. 3. Underdeveloped areas — Social policy — Case studies. I. Title.
HM48.C45   361.6'1   81-20482
ISBN 0-89503-031-4   AACR2

Most of the research discussed in this book was funded by the Taiwanese Family Planning Program and the Population Council during 1963-76. Recent analysis was completed by the author under a Ford and Rockefeller Foundations Award (1979-81). The author thanks his colleagues in Taiwan for their cooperation and encouragement.

This book is dedicated to my parents who continue to wait for me to discover the cure to the common cold.

ISBN 13: 978-0-89503-031-3 (pbk)
ISBN 13: 978-0-415-78605-8 (hbk)

PREFACE

How do you get research results used in an ongoing social service program in a developing country? This book provides some of the answers. Most unusually, it makes its case by weaving theory, methodology, and practice into a rich cultural, political, and bureaucratic context.

As many of you know, the population explosion has touched off another one: the production of books about it. This one, however, stands out as an insightful, perceptive analysis of just why the findings of the researcher are not often integrated into a field-based action program. And, more importantly, it tells us how and why they sometimes are used.

The setting is Taiwan, historically the model family planning program for the 1960's and 1970's. But the implications are international: for developed as well as developing countries. The author knows his material well, having lived what he writes for over ten years in Asia. The case study format is lively and informative.

This important new contribution is *must reading* for anyone involved in social programs. It will be of particular importance to communication and community health education specialists and to planners and applied researchers everywhere. Of special note, it is readable and intended to be discussed thoughtfully in class or in the field.

S. M. Keeny
formerly
Director UNICEF (Asia)
Resident Representative,
The Population Council (East Asia)

CONTENTS

1

AN INTRODUCTION

*The Why and How of this Book ● The Modified Case
Study Format ● Summary of the Case Studies*

THE WHY AND HOW OF THIS BOOK

The purpose of this slender volume is to describe *why* and
how applied research carried out in a national public health program sometimes
influenced program action in the field — and sometimes did not. A number of
modified case studies are presented and analyzed to draw some practical lessons
and to provide a theoretical basis for future program action.

The setting is the Taiwan family planning program. The time period is from
the mid 1960's through the mid 1970's. The focus is on the productive
integration of research findings into community health education programs and
the dissemination of these findings to stimulate other Asian countries at earlier
stages of program planning and implementation.

The viewpoint is that of a former program advisor and community health
educator who spent some ten years on site and observed or participated in the
events described. The results of quantitative research, particularly operations
research and social surveys, recorded documents, and interviews comprise the
methodology used to collect data.

THE MODIFIED CASE STUDY FORMAT

Although there is a growing body of literature on policy
considerations related to population planning, there exist relatively few case
studies. The need for "sophisticated" case studies in the formulation of broad
population policy has been cited by authorities as Berelson [1] among others,

who has stressed the need for case studies in particular settings on the determinants of fertility. The 1973 East West Communication Institute Conference on "Making Population-Family Planning Research Useful" [2] also recommended that more case studies be developed.

There are few case studies on research utilization — certainly not in the population field. Yet, case studies have greatly enriched our understanding of many facets of the overall social development process, particularly our understanding of cultural reaction to introduction of technological innovations in developing countries (e.g., collections of anthropological case studies by E. H. Spicer [3] and Benjamin Paul [4].

The case study approach utilizes the strengths of intensity of approach, detailed formulation of a cultural context, considerable tolerance of the attitude of the investigator to *seeking* rather than *testing* hypotheses, and reliance upon the integrative power of the investigator. Such an approach obviously has some disadvantages as investigators are neither always detached and unbiased observers, nor reporters. This particular case study, however, is somewhat more grounded in empirical, if not objective reality. Grounded in the sense that much of what is analyzed is empirical data and findings from social surveys and experimental and quasi-experimental studies. The case study format allows the introduction of the author's interpretation of these socio-demographic findings in their historic, cultural, bureaucratic and political context. It is hoped that this blending of methodologies of two major approaches to interpreting phenomena will enable the reader to gain a little more insight into both content and process than has been hitherto possible.

SUMMARY OF THE CASE STUDIES

There are eight case studies selected for analysis. They deal both with successes and failures. Emphasis is on analysis of decision-making about research utilization in the economic, educational, bureaucratic, political, cultural, and socio-psychological context in which it occurred. The general "paucity of case materials" [5] on research/knowledge dissemination and utilization (Havelock) and the "absence of case studies" [1] on population policy (Berelson) make this study a unique contribution to scientific knowledge regarding both research utilization and population policy. In addition, considering the generally acknowledged lack of well-designed applied research in community health education, particularly operations research and cost-effectiveness studies, this analysis should also be of considerable benefit to the profession, especially those of us in the West who have a good deal to learn from the experience of the so-called "developing countries."

The first case, *The Case of the Mysteriously Appearing Child*, deals with some of the complexities of applying research findings when:

1. the findings are not focused enough to provide guidelines for action;
2. the organization that wants to win the hearts and minds of the people has yet to convince its own staff;
3. the findings being proposed are too innovative for the political climate of the time; and
4. the organizational network needed to implement the program is a multi-level governmental one and linkage between levels may breach bureaucratic protocols.

The second case, *Sizing Up The Newspapers*, deals with:

1. cost-effectiveness considerations in selecting educational strategies; and
2. tieing in ongoing research with ongoing combined training of community health education and research and evaluation staff to be sensitive to each other's needs.

The third case, *How Not to Price Oral Contraceptives*, is an example of a cleverly-planned operations research project with immense cost-effectiveness considerations. It also demonstrates clearly why research findings are not applied:

1. there were not sufficient funds to implement operationally the results; and
2. a time lag (the findings were not available before program decisions had to be made).

The fourth case, *Pasting Your Umbrella Before the Rain*, reviews the political and cultural barriers to implementing a population education program in a formal school setting. Especially relevant are the ways in which program and research results are given short shrift when program administrators sense an impending threat to their jobs.

The fifth case, *Free Offers for a Limited Time Only*, illustrates the value of involving home-visiting field workers at the township level and the potential consumers of service in a research utilization feedback system. It also demonstrates the need for flexibility in research design and adaptability to evolving field situations. Of special interest to community health educators, it deals with issues of cost-effectiveness.

The sixth case deals with *Today Kaohsiung, Tomorrow Taiwan*. Applied research is used to break the constraints of conservative policy. A mass media demonstration project with carefully thought out objectives is used as a model for a national effort. The importance of trust and close geographic linkage between program administrators and researchers, immediate feedback of results, and building progressively on previous research are stressed.

The seventh case deals with *Incentives: Beyond Family Planning*. Two large-scale non-fertility programs are discussed in terms of how previous research results lead to their implementation. Both of these also demonstrate how continued foreign aid was secured because of a project's innovative and regional implications and the larger political implications thereof. Problems in influencing leaders to take action based on the results of these studies also are reviewed.

The eighth case, *Scientific American goes Asian*, describes the classic Taichung Study. This action-oriented research project helped Taiwan expand to a national family planning program and demonstrated cost-effective ways to implement it. The organization that expedited application of the research to practice and how these results found their way to the desk of most public health and social policy planners and implementors in the developing world are discussed.

A summary of the findings in all the cases is included in Chapter 6. The cases are discussed in terms of research utilization and program implications. Their contributions to a theoretical base for health education practice are presented in Chapter 7.

Four appendices of some practical use follow:

#A – research utilization recommendations of dedicated researchers, communicators and administrators brainstorming on the sands of Waikiki in December of 1974;

#B – a memo presenting a quick and dirty guide to action based on mass media audience surveys;

#C – a memo in dialogue form between a true believer from Taiwan trying to influence skeptics from East and Southeast Asia to use mass family planning mailings; and

#D – the draft grant request used to gain funding for a controversial incentive-oriented non-fertility project (D).

2

CLOSING THE GAP BETWEEN RESEARCH AND PROGRAM ACTION

What Should We Know? • The State of the Art of Research Utilization: A Commentary • Relevant Research Utilization Literature

WHAT SHOULD WE KNOW?

What do we know about the state of the art of research utilization? From the social sciences? From applied fields such as Population? From an applied discipline such as Community Health Education?

Perhaps a better and more selective question for those of us in community health education and applied research and evaluation is "What ought we to know?" This brief chapter synthesizes and tries to summarize some of the relevant literature on research utilization. The relationship to community health education, population studies, and to the subject matter of this book is stated.

THE STATE OF THE ART OF RESEARCH UTILIZATION: A COMMENTARY

Something of what we know about the state of closing the gap between what's known and what's used in programs is summarized below:

1. The body of literature on knowledge utilization and dissemination is growing. Much less, however, exists in the areas of research utilization in such applied areas as rural sociology, education and public health than is desirable. Few reviews attempt to synthesize, classify and disseminate information and fewer still try to develop integrated conceptual models. Rogers [6] and Havelock [5] are notable exceptions in this regard. Their two major reviews attempt to integrate models from a synthesis of

research findings. One is in the area of diffusion of innovations (Rogers) and is drawn from studies primarily in rural sociology, medicine, education and industry. The other is Havelock working at the Center for Research on Utilization of Scientific Knowledge (CRUSK) at the Institute for Social Research, University of Michigan (Ann Arbor). Three models of dissemination and utilization are identified in this synthesis of relevant literature in education and related fields. The three: 1) *Research, Development and Diffusion,* (2) *Social Interaction,* and (3) *Problem Solving,* form the basis for a "linkage model which incorporates important features of all three" (Havelock). This model deserves more attention by health educators and is discussed later in this chapter.

2. Although the overviews of research utilization literature provide examples of "many quantitative research studies, there has been a paucity of case studies as noted by others (Berelson [1], Echols [2], Havelock [5], Cernada and Sun [7]). Without case studies it obviously is difficult to understand events in their cultural, political, or programmatic context.

3. Relatively little other than occasional references to the subject appears in the health education literature about the application of social science theory to the issue of research methodology. There clearly, however, is a theoretical base underlying community health education which could be applied to closing the gap between what is known and what is used in action programs. This volume will attempt to elaborate on some of this theory in examining the case studies presented.

4. Although relatively little has been written in English language health education journals about research utilization, per se, recent notable exceptions include: Reynolds et al. [8], Knutson [9], Khan and Reynolds [10]. Others written by health educators in population-oriented publications, dealing primarily with international programs and in the broad area of Information, Education and Communication (IEC) include Kar [11], Sun and Cernada [7], and Echols [2]. Of these, Khan and Reynolds [10] and Sun and Cernada [7] alone adopt case study formats.

5. The lack of well-designed studies of community health education seems to be a continuing theme in our professional journals. Much of this litany is of serious concern, indeed, for a discipline professing to have a theoretical base and methodologies must demonstrate its worth by application to practice. In an applied field, of course, there is little question about whether there are problems demanding rigorous investigation. As Roberts has said, "health education problems are numerous and varied . . . appearing at many points along the full continuum from health promotion to rehabilitation." [12] The context of family planning programs is no exception.

6. One possible reason for some of our lags in research implementation, of course, lies in our professional training curricula which continue to need strengthening at the graduate levels. Too many with inappropriate or no relevant training are rushing in to attempt research tasks where even angels would fear to tread.

7. Of particular importance in the U.S. is the general lack of knowledge or awareness of the many *planned* attempts to carry out effective health education programs in the so-called "developing" countries. This in itself is a major barrier to research utilization, particularly replication. As Roberts said some time ago:

> Throughout the world, there has been an evident shift toward the use of the educational approach in the prevention and control of health and medical care problems. Combined with this are *planned* attempts to improve the effectiveness of health education, and in some countries, these include formalized efforts to give spur to research and to train research workers. Since health education and its improvement is today of global concern, any examination of research into health educational problems must be developed within a wide perspective, keeping international problems and needs at the forefront while at the same time recognizing various national interests and developments [12, p. 1].

In some respects, health educators have ignored the large body of program implementation, evaluation and applied research existing in developing countries. This ignorance sometimes results from the logistical problems of access to write-ups in journals in other countries and other languages. To some degree, though, it involves a lack of "openness" on the part of U.S. health education leaders who tend to dismiss work done elsewhere as lower standard or at least inapplicable to the U.S. Such egocentric and ethnocentric views are not supported by the facts. For whatever reasons, many developing countries because of their inability to restructure their resources feel that they are unable to afford certain kinds of secondary and tertiary health care and have concentrated on strong preventive and also primary health care programs with varying degrees of community health education components. Few, if any, of these countries implement less than the community health education effort most Western countries have and most have carried out well-designed cost effectiveness/cost benefit studies of these efforts (an area the U.S. is weak on). Furthermore, pragmatic experience has demonstrated that such programs work well in such life-threatening programs as malaria, cholera, TB, etc. This experience has carried over into programs such as maternal and child health, nutrition and family planning.

8. One system to promote research utilization is that developed to support U.S. agricultural efforts by the Cooperative Extension Service (CES). The

purpose is to increase awareness and knowledge levels in farming communities. Government carries out the function but private industry provides the distribution system of commercial products. Although some components of the CES model seem applicable outside of agriculture, the system as a whole is generally considered not to be.

For those who wish to review the literature on research utilization more fully, a selective synthesis of some of the major viewpoints follows. For those who do not, you may move on to our description of the Taiwan setting in which these cases take place.

RELEVANT RESEARCH UTILIZATION LITERATURE

A number of researchers have identified factors which seem to have an effect on whether knowledge gets applied or not. The possible variables governing such utilization in social programs obviously could be innumerable. Even in the area of utilization of research with implications for health education programs, the variables affecting action are many. A brief summary of some of those considered to be important by others, particularly in research related to health education follows.

Havelock, in reviewing some 4,000 studies on knowledge dissemination and utilization, found "remarkable consistency" among them in that certain themes kept coming up. These he summarizes in telegraphic and perhaps oversimplified form as [5, pp. 11-20]:

1. Linkage: The number, variety, and mutuality of Resource System-User System Contacts, degree of inter-relatedness, collaborative relationships.
2. Structure: The degree of Systematic Organization and Coordination of the:
   - resource system
   - user system
   - dissemination-utilization strategy
   - message (coherence)
3. Openness: The Belief that change is desirable and possible. Willingness and readiness to accept outside help. Willingness and readiness to listen to the needs of others and to give help. Social climate favorable to change.
4. Capacity: The capability to retrieve and marshall diverse resources. Highly correlated with this capacity factor are: wealth, power, size, centrality, intelligence, education, experience, cosmopoliteness, mobility and the number and diversity of existing linkages.
5. Reward: The frequency, immediacy, amount, mutuality of, planning and structuring of positive reinforcements.
6. Proximity: Nearness in time, place, and context. Familiarity, similarity, recency.
7. Synergy: The number, variety, frequency, and persistence of forces that can be mobilized to produce a knowledge utilization effect.

A more detailed elaboration presenting these seven factors in terms of how they relate to the knowledge dissemination and utilization process is included in Table 1. This two-dimensional approach illustrates the meaning of each of these seven factors affecting knowledge utilization in terms of four major communication process considerations (*Who* says *What* to *Whom* and *How*).

Havelock reviews three perspectives on knowledge dissemination and utilization:

1. problem solving (P-S);
2. social interaction (S-I); and
3. research, development, and diffusion (R,D+D).

Each of these has major exponents, e.g., P-S has such spokepersons as Ronald Lippit and Goodwin Watson; S-I has Everett Rogers, James Coleman, Elihu Katz; R,D+D has Henry M. Brickell, David Clark. The first focuses on the *user* of the innovation and the outside change agent as a catalyst; the second on the *social environment* of the user; and, the third, on the *resource* person or system. An attempt to fuse these is made with the introduction of a "Linkage" system which emphasizes the user as a problem solver. We will return to these, particularly to Lippit and the P-S model when we review our case study findings in terms of relevant theoretical frameworks.

A useful guidebook to the literature on knowledge transfer and change has been prepared by the Human Interaction Research Institute: *Putting Knowledge to Use: A Distillation of the Literature Regarding Knowledge Transfer and Change* [13]. An illustration of one of the more succinct presentations of concepts follows. To measure whether an organization is "ready" to change by taking up a program and maintaining it, the "AVICTORY" index of "organizational readiness" to change is suggested:

> A = ability to carry out the change (capability, resources, and social costs)
>
> V = values; compatibility with mission or goals
>
> I = ideas or information about the qualities of the innovation (communicability, observability, susceptibility to successive modification, divisibility, reversibility, scientific status)
>
> C = circumstances that prevail at the time (climate of trust, willingness to entertain a challenge)
>
> T = timing or readiness for consideration of the idea; early involvement of potential users
>
> O = obligation or accepted need to deal with a particular problem; relevance, commitment; shared interest in solving recognized problems
>
> R = resistance or inhibiting factors; skill in working through uncertainty and risks
>
> Y = yield or perceived prospect of payoff for adoption; expected reward; belief in the efficiency of the innovation.

Green et al have suggested that such a checklist could be prepared for any particular organization and Green has developed a rating scale for health

Table 1. How General D&U Factors Relate to Process Elements: A Summary

		How General Factors Relate To:		
General D&U Factors	Resource Persons & Systems --- Senders-Disseminators (Who) →	User Persons & Systems --- Consumers-Clients (To Whom) →	Message --- Knowledge Innovation (What) →	Medium --- Channel-Strategy-Tactics (How) →
1. LINKAGE	Collaboration, 2-way Interaction with user and other resources. Simulation of user's problem-solving process.	Collaboration, 2-way Interaction with other users and resources. Simulation of resource system's R&D process.	Relevance to user. Adequacy of derivation and congruence with scientific knowledge.	Allows direct contact. Two-way Interaction.
2. STRUCTURE	Systematic planning of D&U efforts. Division of labor and coordination.	Systematic planning and execution of problem-solving efforts. Integrated social organization of receiver system.	Coherence. Systematic preparation (design, test, package).	Systematic strategy. Timing to fit user's problem-solving cycle.
3. OPENNESS	Willingness to help. Readiness to be influenced by user feedback and by new scientific knowledge. Flexibility and accessibility.	Willingness to be helped, desire to change, to see potential of outside resources. Active seeking and willingness to adapt outside resources.	Adaptability, divisibility, demonstrability of the innovation.	Flexible strategies. Best medium allows internal communications between sender and receiver about the innovation.
4. CAPACITY	Ability to summon and invest diverse resources. ---	Ability to assemble and invest internal resources.	Innovations which result from heavy investment and sophisticated	Capacity of medium to carry maximum information.

	Skill and experience in the helping-resource person role. Power, Capital.	Self-confidence, Intelligence. Amount of available time, energy, capital. Skill, sophistication.	design and development will diffuse more effectively.	Accessibility to maximum number of users in minimum time.
5. REWARD	Reward for Investment in D&U activities in terms of dollars, recognition, knowledge, self-esteem.	Past experience of reward for utilization effort. Return on effort invested in dollars, time, capacity, growth, well-being.	Relative advantage, profitability. Time and labor saving potential. Life-liberty-happiness benefit potential.	Medium which can convey feedback (+ and – reinforcement). Most effective medium has best reward history for sender and receiver.
6. PROXIMITY	Closeness and ready access to diverse resources and to users.	Closeness and ready access to resources, other users. Cosmopoliteness. Psychological Proximity: similarity to, and identification with other users, resources.	Relatedness and congruity with user and user needs. Similarity and congruence with past innovations which the user had adopted. Familiarity to user.	Easily accessible medium, familiar to the user.
7. SYNERGY	The number and diversity of resource persons and change agents who gain access to the user. Continuity, Persistence, and Synchronization of effort.	The number and diversity of different users reached will accelerate the diffusion to social system as a whole.	Redundancy of message. The number and variety of forms in which the message appears and the continuity among forms.	The number and diversity, continuity and persistence of different media used to transmit the message.

SOURCE: Havelock, pp. 11-22.

education in maternal and child health programs [14]. Although the criteria and rating scale are intended for overall evaluation of program structure and process, some criteria in the rating scales could be applied in modified form to a research utilization evaluation of organizational readiness to change.

Rogers in *Communication Strategies for Family Planning*, identifies three broad areas of concern or "social systems" in the process of research findings being integrated into family planning program service in developing countries [15]. These are: the research system, the linking system, and the practitioner system. The barriers to utilization of family planning communication research cited include:

1. the research system providing research results (usually governmental or university) does not recognize the family planning agency practitioner's needs;
2. linkers are not provided to translate practitioner needs to researchers and the program implications of research results to practitioners; and
3. practitioners are often overwhelmed by information overload and cannot concentrate on these particular research results.

Worrall, in his foreword to the Echols report [2] of the results of a 1973 East-West Center Communication Institute Conference on research utilization (*Making Population-Family Planning Research Useful – The Communicator's Contribution*, Honolulu, 1974), noted that the conference focused on two models, marketing and agricultural extension and attempted to "analyze research utilization as a communication process and to see how the insights of communication could be applied to enhance research usability and use." The conference was attended by some thirty researchers, information specialists, program administrators, and representatives of international agencies. A major focus was on the linkage between researcher and practitioner and this subject received the most emphasis, stressing the need to train "linkers" but also to consider "linkage" as a process not just a person.

A number of recommendations were made under four categories: researchers (23), linkage (10), research users or practitioners (4), others (3). Participants were mailed the recommendations and asked to comment on each recommendation's importance, timeliness, audience. A listing of the specific recommendations is attached (see Appendix A).

Kar reviews factors influencing the management and utilization of social science research related to population communication strategies and policies (*Management and Utilization of Population Communication Research*, Honolulu, 1977). His objectives, as he indicates, are not to summarize research findings nor to "develop sets of generalizations or theoretical models." He addresses himself to policy planners and program managers, professionals who use research on the job, and researchers. Twelve factors having a "significant influence on the process of research management and utilization" and which are "amenable to change" are identified and discussed. These include:

1. The causal assumptions used by the planners and the researchers
2. Relative empathy
3. Relative power and control of relevant decisions
4. Perceptions of good and useful research
5. Complexity of the content and semantics
6. The researcher's dilemna[1]
7. Reward system and reference groups
8. Perceptions of effective use of research
9. Relative time perspective
10. Situational factors: contact and accessibility
11. General versus specific applications
12. Feedback and evaluation [11, p. 41].

Others in the health education field have dealt with the topic, albeit not as intensely as with other topics. Knutson discusses the need for expert communication "gatekeepers" and the need to "synthesize, classify and distribute information" if it is to be used [9]. Roberts cites training programs in organized formal settings as necessary if health education research results are to be used in professional practice [12]. This "requires that the profession, the individual practitioner and the researcher" each assume responsibility. Khan and Reynolds indicate that research utilization in developing countries may be even more complex than elsewhere [10].

Others well-known to those trained in health education deal with the importance of improving research utilization. Merton speaks of the "double relevance" of applied research: dual results in "systematic knowledge" and "practical use." [16] Tannenbaum calls attention to the need to "know what the public wants" as the objective of sensible applied research and the key to its getting into practice [17]. Grey speaks consistently to the need to synthesize, classify and distribute information if research results are not to be sterile [18].

This review differs somewhat from the others in that it deals with several case studies and draws from their context some suggestions which may have practical application in the field of family planning as well as other community health education programs. It also discusses these recommendations in terms of theoretical frameworks which underly community health education as a discipline. The degree to which these cases reinforce our present systematic knowledge and theoretical constructs in health education is examined.

It is difficult if not impossible to isolate the consideration of "research utilization" from other more important considerations related to Taiwan's remarkable family planning program. Each case study, or indeed this whole volume for it is itself a case study, deals with social, cultural, political, legal

---

[1] " . . . if a research confirms a planner's beliefs and convictions, it could be perceived as a luxury of questionable value; on the other hand, if a research disproves deeply held convictions upon which major decisions have been based, then not too many planners would be inclined to accept these findings readily." [11, p. 4]

and/or organizational factors involved in the gap between what is known and what is practiced. These factors are intimately related to the macro-level of interrelationships between family planning, health and population policy and overall governmental and private sector social and economic development planning. These include but are not limited to such obstacles to population policy evolvement and implementation as inadequate attention to women's role in development planning (including present legal, cultural, political and bureaucratic handicaps), governmental attitudes toward international opinion and external assistance, and the persistence of pro-natal cultural values (e.g., son preference) in spite of Taiwan's dramatic fertility decline.

3

SETTING: "DON'T FORGET THIS IS A SMALL ISLAND"

"Remember, Taiwan Is a Small Island" • *Factors Facilitating the Taiwan Family Planning Program* • *Population and Family Planning Profile*

"REMEMBER, TAIWAN IS A SMALL ISLAND"

This slogan refers not just to the island's length of only 245 miles and 85 miles across. It also is the "Return to the Mainland" rallying cry reminding its inhabitants that Taiwan is administratively only a province of the Republic of China which has been headquartered temporarily in Taipei for the past thirty years since it left the China Mainland. This "small island" is about ninety miles off the southeast coast of Mainland China. It has one of the highest population densities in the world — more than 1,200 persons per square mile. The eastern half of the island is mountainous with few inhabitants; the western half has several times as many people per square mile (see Figure 1).

This population density and vital political considerations have strongly influenced the relative degree of emphasis the present Government was to place on population programs, particularly fertility control. So long as Mainland China preferred to pretend that it had no population problem, Taiwan maintained a low family planning program profile. So long as the Republic of China (Taiwan) needed collaborative programs with its former partner countries in the United Nations, it had to be particularly cognizant of how the outside world, both developing and developed, viewed its internal and external actions. The family planning program became a model for other developing countries during the 1960's and thousands of workers from Asian countries and others were trained in Taiwan. These and a number of complicated political inter-actions often were extremely important in the evolvement of the Taiwan family

21

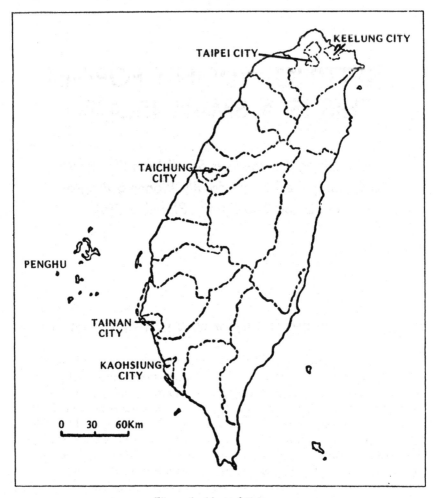

Figure 1. Map of Taiwan.

planning program and its eventual attempts to go beyond health services to in-school population education and broader community participation.

Taiwan achieved a considerable reputation in family planning programming during the 1960's and 1970's. Its record in research utilization is well-known.

Certain countries are especially noted for their high degree of research utilization in the field of family planning; one such nation is Taiwan. A long list of research findings have been implemented in program policies: paraprofessional field workers, diffuser incentives, the coupon system, service fees for private doctors, and non-birth incentives. A basic reason for such research utilization is the close cooperation of researchers and program officials; both are

> housed in the same building, several of the program officials,
> including the director, have Ph.D.'s in demography; and many of
> the researchers have prior experience as program officials. In this
> situation, formally appointed linkers are not needed [15, p. 395].

To some extent, knowledge of the general social, economic, cultural and demographic setting is vital to an understanding of how this research utilization could take place. Following is a brief summary of some of the factors facilitating the growth of the Taiwan family planning program. After this there is a more historical description of the overall population and family planning program evolvement.

FACTORS FACILITATING THE TAIWAN FAMILY PLANNING PROGRAM

A legitimate question is whether the experience of one country is applicable elsewhere. The many countries who have tried to re-invent the wheel again, so to speak, are ample proof that nationalistic pride often dictates to commonsense. To get some overview of some of the factors facilitating Taiwan's family planning program, during the time when the studies in this book took place, a summary description follows.

Factors Facilitating the Taiwan Family Planning Program[1]

Geographical — Taiwan is a small island (245 miles long and 85 miles across at its widest point). Administratively, the island is divided into the Province of Taiwan, and the City of Taipei. The distances between the rural and the urban areas are relatively small.

Cultural — Although Confucianism encourages having sons, it does not explicitly encourage large families; nor does it have any specific doctrine against family planning. Most people believe in a mixture of Buddhism, Taoism, and Confucianism, including ancestor worship. Pure Buddhists comprise less than 10 per cent of the total population; Protestants, about 2 per cent; and Catholics, 1.5 per cent. Religious opposition to family planning is slight.

Linguistic — Although there are two other Chinese dialects, "Taiwanese" and Hakka, most people speak and understand the official language, Mandarin. The written language is the same throughout the country. The media broadcasts in both Mandarin and Taiwanese.

Organizational — There is a strong administrative chain from the National Government in Taipei through the Taipei City and Taiwan Provincial Government

[1] Written by J. F. Tsai.

through twenty counties and small cities, 360 townships, and 6,600 villages. This administrative set-up facilitates the flow of communication in either direction. Family planning organization is centralized within the health networks of both the Province of Taiwan and Taipei City. The program exercises direct control over activities in the field; for example: hiring, training, and dismissal of field workers is centralized at the city and provincial level.

National policy — Taiwan started its program in 1964 without a national policy to support it. This in a way facilitated the initial development of the program in that decisions were made which the government might have considered too rash. Once the acceptability of the program was proven, however, the government became essential for funding.

Vital registration — The Japanese left behind, on this island, a well organized vital registration system which was later strengthened after the Second World War. Almost every birth, death, marriage, and migration is reported and registered at local registration offices. Vital statistics data are, therefore, highly accurate and readily available.

High economic growth — The average rate of economic growth in recent years has been around 8 per cent. This high rate of economic growth has brought some measure of prosperity to the people of the island, has shortened the distance between the rich and the poor, and moreover, has made available more job opportunities, particularly for women. The per capita income in 1970 was US$300 per year; in 1976, close to $1,000.

Education — Free education was extended to nine years in 1968. Enrollment was high — 97.5 per cent during the first six years of schooling (primary), and 74 per cent during the next three years (junior high).

Literacy rate — The literacy rate in Taiwan is one of the highest in Asia: in 1967, in the population over age twelve, it was 88 per cent for male and 67 per cent for female.

Age at marriage — With more young girls in schools and working, the average age at first marriage has been increasing from 18.1 years in 1905, to 20.9 years in 1948, and to 21.6 years in 1967. It may be 23 years by now. Males on the average marry four years later than females.

Good communications network — Communication in terms of transportation is highly advanced in Taiwan. In 1969, the total length of railways was 3,739 km. or 10.5 kilometers for every 100 square kilometers of land area. The total length of highways in the same year was 16,933 kilometers, or 47 kilometers for every 100 square kilometers of land area. From 1946 to 1969 vehicles of all types including motorcycle had increased 1,500 per cent. The population doubled over this same period. Practically every village in Taiwan can be reached by road.

There are ninety-two radio stations, three islandwide TV networks, and thirty-one newspapers. In a survey in 1970, 60 per cent of the women interviewed reported listening to the radio regularly; and 59 per cent reported watching television frequently. On the average, ten persons own one radio set, and forty-two persons own one TV set.

Health services — Health services are readily available and inexpensive. There are 362 health stations in both the Province of Taiwan and Taipei City, averaging one health station per 40,000 population. The doctor population ratio in 1969 was one doctor per 2,400 persons. The death rate began a sharp decline at the end of World War II, and has been below 7 per 1,000 since 1960 and is now at 4.9.

Practice of family planning — The idea of birth control was not new to the people. The Ota ring, another type of IUD, was introduced by the Japanese in the 1930's and has been relatively popular ever since. The practice of female sterilization and induced abortion has been fairly popular even though the latter is illegal and the former's legality has been in doubt.

POPULATION AND
FAMILY PLANNING PROFILE

Size

The earliest dependable report of the inhabitants of Taiwan was written in 1602 by Chen Ti, a Chinese admiral who observed them after pursuing a band of pirates from the mainland of Taiwan. These aboriginal inhabitants are believed to have been of proto-Malayan origin. Only a few Chinese adventurers, small traders, and fishermen came from the mainland, prior to the Dutch colonization starting in 1624. The Dutch encouraged the Chinese to settle and produce sugar for export and rice for local consumption. The Chinese population in Taiwan increased from a few score or hundred in 1600 to an estimated 50,000 by the 1660's. By 1662, the Dutch had been driven out by Koxinga, a royalist of the Ming dynasty, and more migration continued. In the 1680's, there were an estimated 120,000 Chinese. By 1811 there were an estimated two million as immigrants came in greater numbers.[2]

The island was ceded to Japan in 1895. In 1905 the Japanese conducted the first census, estimating a population of 3.1 million. By 1943, the number had increased to almost 6.6 million. When Japan surrendered in 1945, Taiwan was restored to the Republic of China. In 1946, after the out-migration of about

---

[2] These historical data were selected from a number of articles on population growth and social change in Taiwan by the late Shao-hsing Chen, Professor of Sociology, National Taiwan University.

500,000 Japanese, the population was 6,090,860. From 1947 to 1964, slightly more than a million migrated from the mainland. The death rate declined sharply; the population size doubled in only eighteen years, exceeding 12 million in 1964. At the end of 1968 it was 14 million. This rapid growth has made Taiwan one of the world's most densely populated areas.

Growth Patterns

By 1952, the fertility rate had begun to decline. In 1963, a year before the start of the Island-wide family planning program, the crude birth rate was 36.3 per 1,000. The death rate was 6.1. The natural increase rate, 30.2. From 1964, when the family planning program began, the birth rate has declined from 34 to 24 per 1,000 (1979). The population, however, had increased from 12 to 17.5 million and exceeded 18 million in 1981.

Population History

What follows here is largely summarized from a single source and updated as needed [19]. The author recommends that the original source be consulted for further information. This history of population policy evolvement is a useful reference for those readers who wish to better understand the overall context in which the case studies presented took place.

In 1920 Sun Yat-sen, father of the Republic of China, pointed out that if China's population growth rate remained static, as it had for the previous two centuries, China would be taken over by the Western nations. Proponents of Dr. Sun's teaching represented the overwhelming majority for many decades. During those years, population growth was arrested by three natural regulators: disease, famine, and war. By mid-century, however, political stability, agricultural improvement, and the introduction of modern medicine and public health measures in Taiwan had raised the natural increase rate from 20 per 1,000 in 1947 to 38 per 1,000 in 1951. This change prompted the Sino-American Joint Commission on Rural Reconstruction (JCRR) in 1950 to issue a pamphlet on the rhythm method of birth control. The reaction was unfavorable: a petition to the Premier denounced the effort as a Communist plot to weaken the military.

Despite this unpromising beginning, by 1952 JCRR had begun a demographic study partially sponsored by the Rockefeller Foundation and Princeton University. The study clearly indicated that the more children mothers had, the higher the death rate and the more likely the chance of their being placed for adoption. The findings were circulated to government officials and leaders as well as to the public.

In 1954 the China Family Planning Association was begun by a group of individuals in the capital city of Taipei. Their first job was to provide information on infertility and the health value of child spacing during first aid courses given to military dependents.

In 1959, despite difficulties, the Governor of Taiwan agreed to set-up "pre-pregnancy health" (PPH) services at local government health stations. The Governor had become convinced that a reduced population growth rate would not reduce the size of the army for at least 20 years and would definitely be a stimulus to the economy. From 1959 to 1963, 120 of the 361 local health stations added a full-time PPH worker to visit women at home and to provide them with conventional contraceptive methods.

In 1961 the Taiwan Population Studies Center was established in the framework of the Provincial Health Department, with the assistance of the Population Council and the University of Michigan. Its purpose was to undertake surveys and studies on the determinants and consequences of population growth. By releasing its findings it intended to promote better understanding of population problems among administrators and the public.

A year later, the Population Council began the classic experiment in Taichung City (now referred to as the "Taichung Study") to determine what communications approaches reached women best and which contraceptive methods were most desired. The findings showed that the intrauterine device (the Lippes loop) and systematic home-visiting were the best approaches.

In 1963 the newly-appointed Health Commissioner extended the family planning action-study program beyond Taichung City. The following year, K. T. Li, Minister of Economic Affairs, arranged to provide US$1.5 million in local currency from a special account derived from US counterpart funds to conduct a five-year family planning program. The main reason for his action was the recognition of the economic value of lowering the rate of natural increase from 3 per cent to less than 2 per cent.

As early as 1964 the Ministry of Interior had formed a Population Policy Study Committee. Since there were politically strong members opposed to any policy of regulating growth, no recommendations were made. In June 1966 the new Minister reorganized the committee, effectively excluding opponents. Twelve months later two documents were produced: (1) a set of regulations governing the implementation of family planning in Taiwan and (2) an outline of population policy for the Republic of China. These were submitted to the Executive Yuan (Cabinet) for adoption.

In May 1968, on the opening day of the first East Asian Population Conference in Taipei, the government announced its approval of the family planning program regulations. This promulgation effectively legitimized what had been previously an unofficial family planning program, which had been extended throughout the island from 1964 to 1968 [19].

Program Update

Taiwan's exceptional family planning efforts, begun in 1964 on an island-wide basis, have been instrumental in lowering its natural increase rate from 30 per 1,000 in 1963 to 19 by 1973 [20]. This drop from 3 per cent to less than 2 per cent in a decade had been a remarkable achievement. The island, however, remains faced with the perplexing reality that in spite of intensive educational and service inputs, the crude birth rate has been stalled at 23 per 1,000 since 1973 (rising to 25.9 in 1976 and down again to 23.8 in 1977). The present three-year Family Planning Promotion Plan, which is part of the ongoing National Six-Year Economic Development Plan, calls for a lowering of the population increase rate to 1.6 per cent by 1982. Such an achievement seems a difficult task with the rapidly increasing numbers of younger women who are entering marriagable ages. In addition to its efforts to shift emphasis to promoting later marriage, earlier use of contraception, and birth spacing among younger women, the government also has begun to consider relaxing present legal restrictions relating to induced abortion, including review of the present Criminal Law Code, and establishment of an Eugenic Protection Law [21].

4

RESEARCH UTILIZATION IN AN ONGOING FAMILY PLANNING PROGRAM*

Introduction • Summary of Factors Favorable to Research Utilization • Reasons Why Some Research Was Not Utilized • Some Analysis of Favorable Factors • Dissemination of Results Internationally

This chapter deals with why the applied research carried out in the Taiwan family planning program facilitated the planned program of social change — both in the productive integration of research findings into community health education action programs and in the dissemination of these ideas to other Asian countries. A summary of the factors that assisted or hindered research utilization and an analysis of some of the especially favorable factors in the Taiwan situation are presented. The viewpoint presented is that of the Taiwan Institute of Family Planning Director and his former resident program advisor. Eight case studies follow this chapter.

INTRODUCTION

There is considerable consensus among field practitioners of the art of research utilization that its state is far less advanced than social development planners would like [22–24]. This chapter explains why the Taiwan program of family planning has claimed to be a notable exception — both in integrating its research findings into health education action programs and in disseminating these ideas to other Asian countries during the late 1960's and early 1970's where they have found replication in studies and application to virtually all national family planning programs in the region [25].

* Written by George P. Cernada and T. H. Sun.

As is widely known, Taiwan's natural increase rate dropped from 3 per cent to less than 2 per cent in a decade (i.e., from 30 per 1,000 in 1963 to 19 by 1973), partially as a result of the intensive family planning program effort [26]. The major focus of this chapter is on the reasons why the extensive applied research carried out as part of this program had an effect. It would be less then candid, though, not to admit that Taiwan has had as many failures as successes in its applied research. Because Taiwan learned from some of its mistakes, this chapter calls the reasons for them to your attention. Therefore, the outline for this discussion is as follows:

1. *Summary of Factors Favorable to Research Utilization*;
2. *Reasons Why Some Research Was Not Utilized*; and
3. *Some Analysis of Favorable Factors.*

Applied research in the Taiwan family planning program grew from 1963 through the late 1970's from an early concentration on improving the effectiveness (social and cost) of contraceptive services to a later focus on expanding health education and communication approaches — from only face-to-face home visiting, to the use of mass media, to ways of reaching the increasing numbers of younger women whose fertility rates were not dropping [27].

Program experience showed that the needed population changes went far beyond family planning program activities, and community health education efforts expanded to include trying to identify the economic, psychological, and societal values placed upon children; the obstacles to parents' understanding of the advantages of a two-child family; the nature of son preference; educational approaches to newlywed and newly engaged couples; and the interrelationships of population planning to other broader-based social and economic development planning [28]. Perhaps the most significant outcome of this continuing research has been the growing awareness of the complexity of the issues that once were dealt with so simplistically.

SUMMARY OF FACTORS FAVORABLE TO RESEARCH UTILIZATION

Factors which facilitated Taiwan utilizing its research in its population and family planning program, and particularly in the health education and communication components, include:

1. translating program needs into researchable projects, interpreting research findings into simple step-by-step action program changes, and using help from resident/foreign advisors in doing so;
2. adhering to the basic assumption that research is intended to improve the continuing program and to aid in planning future operations which will benefit the consumer;

3. training both program administrators and applied researchers to take on the role of the other and to gear into the other's value system;

4. the accumulation of continually evaluated experience over more than a decade [29] and its cumulative effect on growth of awareness of the complexity of this area of planned social change;

5. an unusually rich flow of vital data and program information, fed back and forth between the program headquarters and the field to help pinpoint research needs, the relatively small size of the island, the already existing well-developed communications network, and the exceptionally accurate vital data available facilitated progress;

6. centralized administrative arrangements: both the research and evaluation and the action program implementation for the most part have been the responsibility of one agency under one directorship and under one roof — this organization has been flexible enough to change to meet consumer needs and program goals;

7. training research staff to be sensitive not only to research methodology but to the need for practical application so that their value system is more in accord with that of program staff (more still needs to be done);

8. training administrators how to interpret research findings and to integrate them into policy decisions and program implementation (as much more needs to be done);

9. flexibility in research funding and research operations so that early stages in exploratory studies can be focused to meet program needs;

10. theoretical and methodological approaches which fitted the action program problem, rather than the opposite (this has meant an awareness that most approaches and research models have far too many limitations to be applied consistently in the field);

11. designing field experiments and pilot projects to demonstrate the means of breaking out of the bounds of current program practice; field observation, service statistics, and results of large social surveys have helped pinpoint some of these demonstration needs;

12. encouraging research and program staff to solve problems as a team and to be proud of their achievement — with incentives added, such as providing publication vehicles and salary supplements; and

13. recognition of mistakes and learning from them as well as from successes; evaluators have continued to objectively evaluate their own research and to invite and listen to outside criticism.

REASONS WHY SOME RESEARCH WAS NOT UTILIZED

The authors have identified several factors which hindered research use in Taiwan's program. These include, but are not limited to, the following.

1. findings calling for changes were interpreted to be in conflict with government regulations;
2. no available budgets to implement findings;
3. time lag: by the time findings were available and translated for program use, the program was ahead of the study;
4. the research project began without sufficient involvement of the staff who would have to implement the findings;
5. armchair research — not enough relationship to the situation in the field it was designed to solve;
6. the study methodology was questionable;
7. the study objectives were inadequately defined;
8. the findings were not conclusive enough to justify program change;
9. the island-wide social survey needs assessment approach (stressed during the last half of the 1960's) should have been preceded by more exploratory work or followed up more in depth to pinpoint certain trends among groups;
10. the research was urged upon the unit by outside agencies and interest in results was mostly theirs;
11. the needed change might have thrown another aspect of the program out of balance;
12. findings might have caused someone to lose face;
13. the manner in which the findings were presented to the program staff violated protocol or was threatening;
14. the applied research project represented only the researcher's interest; and
15. the research did not gear into the broader scope of social change occurring at the time.

SOME ANALYSIS OF FAVORABLE FACTORS

Organization

The Research and Evaluation Unit was located in the Committee on Family Planning of the Taiwan Provincial Health Department, which had responsibility for promoting the family planning program in Taiwan Province. It evolved in 1969 from its predecessor unit, the former Taiwan Population Studies Center, which was started in 1961. It is presently the Taiwan Provincial Institute of Family Planning. Its strength in terms of research utilization lies in the following:

1. the organization evolved over more than a decade; the divisions of labor, staffing, and functions were adjusted continually to meet the program's evaluation needs;

2. the family planning program agency contains both the evaluating and the implementing units at the same level; they are in the same building – this eliminates many jurisdictional squabbles and lessens communication problems;

3. excellent sample social survey facilities have been developed, including an unusually good sampling framework (developed in consultation with the University of Michigan), strong interviewing team and field interviewing supervision, good coding personnel, an efficient data processing unit and experienced and capable research staff;

4. the Institute's director has had extensive experience and training in research and evaluation and works closely with these units;

5. close relationship with other organizations such as the former Joint Commission on Rural Reconstruction and the Council for International Economic Cooperation and Development (locally), and the Population Council and the University of Michigan Population Studies Center (in the United States) increased the opportunity for outside inputs of ideas for new directions and critical reactions to projects being implemented during the 1960's and 1970's;

6. the autonomy of the evaluation group is maintained by having separate sections which are able to be reasonably objective – these form three of the six units at headquarters and a third of the professional staff: one emphasizes intermediate and longer-term studies, the second focuses on analysis of input-output data, the third does the processing (since the first two must keep close track of field programs, there is considerable feedback into and from the action units – education, supervision, and planning); and

7. the field network stretches throughout the island: the field supervisory teams are able to locate problem areas as they arise, and also to transfer the findings for implementation.

Staff

The following are strengths:

1. meetings are held weekly by program and research units to review activities: each division has a quarterly work plan (specifying weekly activities) distributed to all others – this helps develop a common value system in respect to sharing responsibility for a good overall job;

2. there is considerable teamwork and a problem-solving orientation developed on the strength of having overcome many obstacles, some through applied research efforts;

3. an education evaluation committee reviews communication needs; both education and research staff discuss problems and how to solve them; the

limitations of both program and evaluation units become clearer so that realistic demands are made; a single problem is approached by several staff from different viewpoints; process as well as task receives emphasis so that staff can develop;

4. program progress and interim reports on research are circulated regularly so that each staff person is able to get an idea of what is going on in the program as a whole;

5. senior research staff have received graduate training abroad, usually only after several years of working experience; by the time they go abroad they have a feeling of how research helps the program and are able to view coursework in terms of on-the-job applicability; their overseas training emphasizes quantitative measurement but is basically in social sciences: major in sociology (Michigan), demography (University of Pennsylvania) for example; senior program staff who work with them are trained abroad in health education and communication, also only after on-the-job experience;

6. working assignments are arranged so that each person has responsibility for at least one study on his own — studies are matched with staff interests, training, and experience, with individual growth in mind as well;

7. co-authorship of papers is encouraged: in a mimeographed "Interim Reports" series, a "Working Paper" series (in conjunction with the University of Michigan Population Studies Center) and in local and foreign journals, (e.g., *Studies in Family Planning*) — these papers provide a sense of satisfaction and pride; and

8. fellowship support for graduate training abroad is an incentive for recruiting staff as well as for maintaining them — more support sources are needed now.

Funding

1. much of the research funding, particularly for more innovative projects which local sources would not support, was available from external sources — gradually, local sources have taken over this function.

2. Because of a long-time association with one external assistance agency, the Population Council, needed funding for research and fellowship study abroad dovetailed nicely with other program funding sources.

3. Considerable flexibility in the use of outside funding for research projects was possible and encouraged whenever interim findings indicated needed changes in research and evaluation projects.

4. Salary supplements have been available to recruit promising evaluation staff candidates and to maintain a nucleus of key experienced research staff. These came first from external sources and later from local support.

Determination of Research Needs

Research needs were defined primarily by potential program applicability. This was possible because the evaluation and research unit was integrated into the overall action program organization. Most of the more than 100 formal studies carried out tried to answer questions posed by program problems. Where possible, evaluation was built into continuing program activities – e.g., systematic collection of service statistics, measures of program input and output, supervisory observations in the field, and special projects carried out by the operational divisions of the Institute of Family Planning.

Some strengths include the following.

1. Crude birth rate and contraceptive acceptor goals were set. Whenever program obstacles were encountered, the Research and Evaluation Unit was asked to help find out how to overcome these. This meant that research priorities focused largely on problems related to *consumers* of service or program implementors, not just the interests of research (or action program) personnel.

2. Priorities for research were based on potential for program implementation and on researchability. The choice for the most part rested with a director sensitive to both research and program activities. Resident advisors also played a vital role in helping to identify consumer needs and in translating program needs into applied research study designs.

3. There was a continuing two-way flow of communication between the field and headquarters: service statistics, input-output measures, regular headquarters meetings, regular field staff meetings, and meetings of field with headquarters staff. These have helped determine and clarify research needs. The home-visiting field workers were usually the first to learn from people in the villages what was going wrong or right in the program.

4. The continued difficulties of getting adequate funding (due to a lack of Government policy through 1968) meant greater attention to *cost-effectiveness* studies of all sorts: in mailings, in home visits vs. group meetings, and so on. The series of cost-effective studies is probably one of the most extensive of its kind and is widely documented in international journals [7, 30–36].

5. The multiple agencies which served as sources of local funding demanded early that the research unit show results by evaluating the effectiveness of the program or else lose its funding. This was a constant incentive to practical application during the early years of the operation.

6. Most research has been applied but not all has been short-term. There was considerable emphasis on intermediate and long-term work (particularly experimental approaches – the educational savings plan, maximum contraceptive acceptance plan, spacing incentive approach) [32, 37] when it became apparent from research findings that goals could

not be realized without influencing social change more dramatically than by offering only contraceptive-oriented service and education.

Using Results

1. Field experiments and pilot projects have been designed to clearly illustrate the value of breaking out of current program practice limits. The excellent survey facilities have been used to provide baselines for these pilot approaches. Many times these demonstration projects have been suggested by field observation and the results of larger social surveys.

2. An early warning system is used to build in self-evident feedback systems to increase the evaluative component so that failures, successes, and problems can be identified early (e.g., with mailing campaigns [34], the coupon system [38], free offers [36, 38, 39].

3. Field and program staff who need the research results are involved early. They have requested solutions to problems. They help plan the study to the extent of their research capabilities; they are kept informed of activities; they revise questionnaires. When results come in they participate in analysis where possible. Their skepticism of results keeps research staff alert.

4. Final decision-making based on whether to take on research and to apply findings has rested for the most part with a director who has been sensitive both to research and program activities.

5. Resident foreign advisors were important in helping translate research findings into program implementation for the consumer's satisfaction and helping maintain continuing liaison between program and research staff. An important aspect has been capsulizing research results into simplified steps that are feasible in an action setting.

6. Early analysis reports are mimeographed and distributed for discussion and comment.

7. Field staff are briefed thoroughly about results affecting their work.

8. Linkage between research and program has been cumulative: program needs are met not only by new research projects but also by examining the bank of accumulated knowledge of many previous studies. Applied results of one study lead to feedback and re-examination of the newly acquired and older accumulated data. These may lead to a new study. Many action results were possible because they were supported by findings from more than one research project.

9. The continuing liaison between program and research staff is assisted by such groups as the education evaluation committee who plan the IEC program in terms of what the accumulated body of knowledge is, the program's goals, the staffing, limited funding, and limitations of various IEC approaches.

DISSEMINATION OF RESULTS INTERNATIONALLY

The Taiwan program was of special interest to the international community for more than a decade. Various aspects of its program have been incorporated into other national programs in Asia (Indonesia, the Philippines, Thailand, and South Korea), e.g., the methods of selection, training and types of home-visiting field workers, the use of targets, diffuser incentives, the coupon system to quickly get data on numbers and characteristics of recent contraceptive acceptors, regular sample follow-up surveys of acceptors, how to set up small pilot studies to get quick results [40].

This diffusion of Taiwan's experience seems to be due to a number of factors: the program was the earliest "successful" one in the area [31]; the results were widely publicized as the program progressed; the quality of vital data was exceptional; and thousands of Asians visited the program to learn about specific aspects both before their countries began programs and while they were starting them. Moreover, both the Population Council and the University of Michigan Population Studies Center disseminated considerable publicity about the program among other countries and in the U.S. The Council and other international population agencies provided funding to key leaders in programs (or potential programs) to visit Taiwan. There was extensive documentation of program activities — particularly many well-documented "demonstration-type" studies. And both resident foreign advisory and program operation staff from Taiwan have gone to other assignments on population in Asia and other countries and applied this experience.

Strengths include:

1. The government has a policy of encouraging aid to other developing countries — e.g., study of land reform and agricultural development — and therefore helps support activities of the Chinese Center for International Training in Family Planning. The Center draws on Institute programs and research staff on a part-time basis. This arrangement assured the several hundred visitors from Asian countries annually of up-to-date simplified summaries of research and program results. Many of these countries have adapted aspects of Taiwan's approaches to their programs.

2. Extensive documentation helps other local scholars and government planners get a firmer baseline before carrying out their own studies. Frequent visits have led to cooperative research efforts to get at problems such as son preference that may require methodological approaches in which Institute staff have less skill.

3. Selected mailing lists drawn from interested visitors allow related materials to be sent intermittently to key program and research staff, particularly in Asia.

4. Findings are frequently simplified and tailor-fitted to different audiences:

local and national economic planners, field staff, other program staff, funding agencies, university students, and international visitors.

5. Important studies are quickly written up and sent to journals which get them to an interested and large audience quickly — e.g., *Studies in Family Planning*. United States university and local resident advisory staff were helpful in expediting this process.

6. An annotated bibliography of some 300 key articles is available [41]. A summary of more than 100 studies provides a brief description, findings and references [42]. Simplified chartbooks provide graphic illustrations of the findings of key new studies and their relation to one another in terms of the population problem in Taiwan.

7. Collections of articles on specific topic areas are assembled — for example, forty-seven recent articles on IEC activities [43].

8. Interim reports, bimonthly, quarterly, semi-annual and annual reports on program and research progress and quarterly program plans help keep staff alert to developments and help maintain a production schedule. The several funding agencies also can keep abreast.

Conclusion

As Taiwan's population program has shifted emphasis to deal with promoting later marriage, earlier use of contraception, birth spacing, and interdisciplinary approaches to understanding the cultural role of son preference and related social and economic development considerations such as increased employment opportunities for women, it has continued this trend of sharing its thinking. Although the program, like the Island as a whole, has become largely independent of international aid and resident foreign advisory services, it still nurtures working relationships with many professionals in Asia and abroad, particularly in joint applied research activities. It also continues to provide short-term training through the Chinese Center for International Training in Family Planning,[3] and disseminates program information through mailings of progress reports to colleagues in Asia and through active participation in the International Committee for Applied Research in Population[4] established by Asian family planning program leaders in the 1970's for this purpose.

ACKNOWLEDGEMENTS

This chapter covers the work of the Taiwan Provincial Institute of Family Planning and its predecessors, the Committee on Family Planning and Taiwan Population Studies Center of the Taiwan Provincial Health Department.

[3] J. F. Tsai, Director, CCITFP, P.O. Box 112, Taichung, Taiwan, 400, R.O.C.
[4] Program leaders in a number of Asian programs, e.g., Bangladesh, Indonesia, South Korea, Thailand.

Special thanks are due to the present and former staff of these agencies for their contributions and also to such key figures as Minister K. T. Li, B. Berelson, Y. C. Chen, Dr. L. P. Chow, O. D. Finnigan, R. Freedman, R. Gillespie, V. Jamieson, A. Hermalin, Dr. S. C. Hsu, L. Kincaid, Dr. T. C. Hsu, Dr. H. T. Hu, Dr. T. Y. Lee, S. M. Keeny, Dr. J. LeComte, L. Lu, Dr. J. Y. Peng, Dr. J. Russell, Everett Rogers, L. Springfield, J. Y. Takeshita, Dr. C. M. Wang, R. Worrall, and Dr. C. H. Yen.[5]

[5] This chapter is a reprint of the article from the *International Quarterly of Community Health Education* (2:1, 1981). It is an abridged version of a longer monograph published by the East-West Center (East-West Communication Institute Paper, No. 10, 1974).

5

CASE STUDIES

EIGHT CASES AND
DISCUSSION SUGGESTIONS

#1 — THE CASE OF THE MYSTERIOUSLY
APPEARING CHILD

*Summary • Calendar of Events • Results • The Mysteriously
Appearing Child • Commentary • Suggestions for Discussion*

SUMMARY

This case study is a bit of a fisherman's tale of the big one
that got away. In retrospect, its dimensions loom larger in the author's mind
than perhaps the circumstances of the time warranted. On the other hand, the
episode described remains as a significant symbol of the immense gap between
what is known and what can be done in a bona fide health education program
and of how little we really know about how to translate research findings into
program action. We are often handicapped by inadequate theoretical
orientations from social psychology, questionable methodologies (e.g., KAP
surveys) and a lack of significant understanding of how research fits into the
organizational structure outside our agency or the broader spectrum of social
change where it ultimately must be dealt with or not by the public.

This short vignette began in 1973 when the author came across an article on
philatelic progress on population. The article noted that since 1965 a large
number of developing countries had issued postage stamps as an educational
component in their family planning programs. All but Taiwan and Indonesia
were similar in that they depicted parents and two children. Golda surmised

that in these two countries, "the slogan 'stop at two' did not influence the design of these stamps" since the Taiwan and Indonesia stamps "each depict three" children [44]. As right as the author was in noting the discrepancy, she was wrong in assuming that the Taiwan design was not influenced by the "Stop at Two" slogan. The story of how this postage stamp finally managed to be pasted onto three million envelopes in 1970 may help development planners and educators better understand the complexity of the educational problems involved and the intricacies of political and administrative logistics in applying research in a family planning program in a developing country.

CALENDAR OF EVENTS

Mid-1964

From mid-1964 when the Taiwan family planning program became active on an island-wide scale, the educational approach was primarily home visits to mothers by full-time fieldworkers. Leaflets and pamphlets were provided as were a limited number of posters. Mass media use, however, was limited by lack of a government policy supporting the program. Even the fieldworkers were euphemistically called "pre-pregnancy health" (or PPH) workers.

1967

Program personnel, though, were aware of the possibilities of using a family planning postage stamp, as suggested in 1967 in memos to the family planning program director stressing the value of moving beyond the health areas. The earlier Korean "Family Planning Month" stamp (mid-1965) had been called to the attention of key staff as correspondence among family planning administrators and local foreign resident advisors in both Taiwan and Korea was extensive during this pioneering period. Administrators also were aware of the high literacy, the high volume of letters mailed, and a postal network that could get a special delivery letter to virtually anywhere in the island in a day. Furthermore, Island-wide KAP surveys had shown that the "average" ideal number of children among married women was four and statistical projections predicted a demographic explosion. No action was taken, though, because:

1. as yet there was no *official* government policy supporting the family planning program;
2. the few agencies involved in the family planning program were health agencies — with little political power;
3. the family planning agency had no contact with the Ministry of Communications which would have to sanction the issuing of a stamp to its National Directorate of Posts; and

4. the program existed at the Taiwan Provincial Government level and most staff were unclear about what the policy of the national government (the Republic of China) was.

May 1968

An official policy supporting the family planning program was announced by the Vice-President and Premier at the opening of the East Asian Population Conference in Taipei in May 1968. This opened the possibility for use of agencies other than health.

May 1969

A list entitled "What Other Agencies Can Do to Help Lower the Birth Rate" was prepared to supplement a list of what public health agencies planned to do to expand activities. After several months of deliberation, it was decided that in order to get action at the national level (the family planning program was conducted at the Taiwan province-level), the resident foreign advisory staff should submit the list to the then Minister of Economic Affairs, a long-time supporter of the family planning program. The list involved more than a dozen agencies at the national and provincial levels, and actions requested ranged from integrating population education into the school curriculum through expanding family planning training for military recruits and reservists. The stamp was only one of many activities in the public information sphere.

August 1969

With the backing of the Provincial Health Commissioner, the list was sent directly to the Minister of Economic Affairs by the local resident foreign advisory staff, thus bypassing what might have involved circuitous routing indeed to get from the unofficial Family Planning Institute of the Taiwan Provincial Health Department to the Taiwan Provincial Government and then to the various National Ministries.

The Minister referred the suggestions to the National Cabinet (Executive Yuan) for consideration and the Cabinet referred them to the Ministry of Interior to discuss appropriate responsibility and possibilities of implementation.

September 1969

The Population Policy Committee of the Ministry of Interior (MOI) met on September 8 to discuss implementing the list of suggested ways other government agencies could help curb population growth. The MOI's Population Division and their Health Office, the Executive Yuan, the Council for

International Economic Cooperation and Development, the Taiwan Provincial Health Department, the Taiwan Provincial Institute of Family Planning, the Taipei City Health Bureau, the National Defense Ministry, the Ministry of Communications, the National Directorate of Posts, the Ministry of Finance, the Joint Commission on Rural Reconstruction, the National Office of Information, and the Ministry of Education were represented. The foreign advisor was an observer.

Little League Influence

The National Directorate of Posts was asked to do two things:

1. use a postal franking device to stamp all letters: "Practice Family Planning"; and
2. issue a postage stamp advocating family planning.

The proponents went to the meeting hoping to get item one, but doubtful about two. To their delight, both were approved, after an amusing exchange which illustrates the need for foreigners to keep abreast of current social developments. When the postage stamp topic was introduced, the postal official was quick to tell us that he sympathized, but that the stamp was not a likely possibility. Under current regulations a regular stamp issue could not be released; only a special commemorative stamp would be possible. Alas, the waiting list for commemoratives was at least two years long. What could be done? The observer took this occasion to facetiously ask who was their sports consultant who had predicted so far in advance that the Little League World Championship would be won by Taiwan! After all, the stamps celebrating the victory had been out within weeks after the series. The postal official joined the group in laughing and after some discussion agreed that family planning was in the long run as important as the Little League victory — even if it was a first world championship.

RESULTS

October-November 1969

The Executive Yuan reviewed and approved the list of actions that the various government agencies had agreed to at the September 8 meeting. Various agencies were requested to implement the plans. Family Planning Institute staff were asked to prepare a draft stamp and a postal franking device slogan. The postal franking device, "Practice Family Planning" was stamped on all mail at all post offices for a one-month period from mid-November to mid-December, 1969.

The stamp proved to be more difficult. The major program slogan was "3-3-3-33" (after marriage postpone the first child three years; wait three years between children; have only three; stop at age thirty-three), but younger innovative staff decided two might be better since their demographic research showed that the birth rate was not declining fast enough and there was an upcoming cohort of increasing numbers of younger couples (postwar baby boom). Discussion focused on whether two or three children ought to be illustrated on the stamp. The question was "if four is the ideal desired number for most couples, should you push for closer — three — or go further — two?" "Wasn't two a better ideal demographically?" Also, there was interest in moving away from son preference. At the time, those advocating two cited the demographic need — to achieve a zero-growth rate of population by the year 2030 meant bringing the net reproductive rate to one (i.e., approximately 2.1 children) by 1978. Nobody mentioned one child seriously; none, as might be expected, was not likely to be mentioned. The more practical-minded contended that three was closer to the real present ideal and hence more likely to be acceptable to people since parents would be strongly ego-involved on such an issue. The initial planners, however, settled upon two.

December 1969

Draft postage stamp designs with the two child theme were sent to an intermediary agency, the Joint Commission on Rural Reconstruction (JCRR), for submission and discussion with the National Directorate of Posts. The JCRR had filled this role of "midwife" or "go-between" before and in this case the several hours train ride between Taichung, the provincial capital (where the family planning program was then headquartered) and Taipei, the national capital (where the Postal Directorate was) and the difference in administrative levels (provincial and national) influenced the decision to use an intermediary.

During the negotiations, it was agreed to print 2.5 million of the NT$1 issue — which was the postage rate for a first-class letter. This was important to get a wider distribution of the stamp. Another 0.5 million of an NT$4 stamp would be issued as well — partly for international use and also for packages. The stamp's message was kept as free from political repercussions as possible. It stated simply, "Family Planning." The picture depicted a "model" happy family.

THE MYSTERIOUSLY APPEARING CHILD

November 11, 1970

The day the stamp was finally issued, our mystery begins. A third child had mysteriously appeared to join the two proposed by the Institute of Family

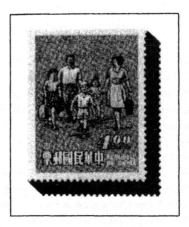

Figure 2. Family planning postage stamp.

Planning design. The family planning program staff were disappointed; the younger innovators appeased only by the fact that one stamp (NT$4) showed two girls and one boy (ideal size included a two-son preference in Taiwan). What happened between the design and the issue is still unsettled. It was not until many years later that this author learned from the JCRR "go-between" just how the third child entered into the picture, but the details are as yet unclear. What seems evident in retrospect is that not enough education was provided on the value of the "two-child ideal" to convince even the proponents of the stamp to carry through the theme. In fact, little had been done to educate most of the public health staff. (See Figure 2.)

One handicap in applying research was the shaky theoretical base in social psychology on which it rested. Whether two children ought to have been illustrated depends upon a better understanding of the relationship between communication distance and opinion change than present research can provide us, as well as a better understanding of the dynamics of the situation from this point onward. One social psychology consideration which seems important is that: if the issue of number of children is ego involving (as would be suspected), and the communicator has less credibility (little is known in this respect), the communicator ought to take a less extreme position, i.e., push for three rather than two children. But since so many of the social-psychological findings on communication and persuasion are based upon small samples of selective audiences (the traditional college sophomores), they are open to question. Nevertheless, a good argument can be made for pushing three children rather than two when an ideal size is four. On the other hand, there is the problem later of how to shift from three to two — still unanswered! For specific individuals or groups known to have an ideal of three (mostly younger), the answer is easier but expensive: pitch a special campaign to them.

COMMENTARY

All the research in the world is not going to solve a practical problem if the persons who must implement it are not involved in the early thinking and planning related to that research. Over a long period of time the "go-between" for the family planning program with the national level had become disenchanted with research for its own sake. A field man by nature, he believed too much program attention was going to research which often would not be applied and sometimes was more to the benefit of foreign institutions than Taiwan's. When the program began its transition to a "two-child" theme, he expressed considerable concern that the change was too abrupt and that the credibility of the program (long a public advocate of "three children") would be damaged. In the final analysis, the "go-between" decided that it would be in the program's longer-term interests not to press for a "two-child" theme in the postage stamp since the issuing of the stamp was itself a major concession and the legislators who would review the issue (and themselves had many children) might be aroused. Indeed, he may have been right. And so, considerations about research findings were relegated to minor factors in what was a *political* policy decision.

In terms of research utilization, the failure to involve a wider circle of the overall organizational forces earlier was a major handicap (see Figure 3).

Reliance on a research base which was open to many questions also was a problem. It would have been useful at the time to have had the kind of inter-disciplinary studies on son preference and economic and non-economic values placed on children which were carried out in the mid-1970's. Timing, of course, was a major factor: findings were too innovative to be accepted at that point when there was considerable concern by the Government that fertility regulation programs maintain a low profile.

It is important to note, though, that the postage stamp did serve useful educational ends for it:

1. provided a first example of how communication agencies other than public health could be used to promote family planning;
2. had high public visibility as the opinion of the government and is believed to have stimulated various government departments to help the program; and
3. boosted local family planning morale, particularly fieldworkers'.

Of some importance also was the program's use of the foreign advisor as a link or liaison to agencies at several levels of government. When family planning and public health staff at the Provincial level could not get to decision-makers at the national level, they decided to enlist their program advisors to serve as "floating advisors" and "linkers" to organizations where formal linkage was impossible. This linkage broadened gradually over the later years from policy

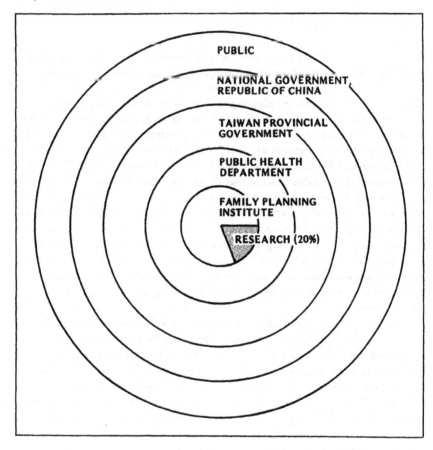

Figure 3. Inter organizational chart: family planning research.

implementation to establishing ties to conduct joint research with other institutions.

Linkage between governmental agencies at various organizational and hierarchical levels is difficult to achieve. It is possible, however, to locate individuals who because of family ties, social standing, political memberships or even affiliation with a supra-national or international agency may be allowed to provide liaison on an inter-governmental agency level. Such linkage can help bring *useful* research findings to the attention of program implementors and policy makers.

Both research and program implementation staff need to understand and believe what they are trying to educate the public about. In-service staff education is vital.

There appears to be far more public concern about the expertise and trustworthiness of provision of services and "educational" output by governmental programs than there is applied research on source credibility. Without this knowledge, some programmatic actions lack direction.

There is an appropriate and inappropriate time for any educational intervention. It is easier to determine the latter. Both researchers and program staff need to be more appreciative of when a program policy maker or chief executive needs to listen to the louder voice of higher-level bureaucrats or the public. Both parties need to keep abreast of just what the political, bureaucratic and public atmosphere is conducive to in the same manner that they keep posted on research findings or other bureaucratic events.

SUGGESTIONS FOR DISCUSSION

1. Isn't more research needed into the values area? In what ways can the two-child ideal of ZPG be more than a slogan or litany in developing countries? Should it be more?

2. Is son preference really economically necessary to parents in developing countries? What more can be done to find out about cultural aspects of son preference?

3. How can a country prepare itself for a transition in an educational campaign — from promotion of an ideal desired number of three children to only two?

4. Are any programs educating their own staff *before* trying to reach the public (on the two-child ideal and son preference)? Can you think of parallel situations in U.S. programs, e.g., cancer control, mental health, others?

5. Given the little known about the economic and noneconomic values of children, would it have been likely that there was enough "Content" available to convince people about a two-child ideal anyway?

6. Would having had two children on the stamp with a statement such as "Family Planning" been understood to be advocating "only two" anyhow?

7. Shouldn't there have been a pretest of the stamp? (A posttest of whether it was seen was included in an island-wide KAP survey — but not until 1973.)

8. In general, what kind of research do you think is likely to influence national leaders? How have programs brought findings to the attention of the leaders?

9. What do you see as the ethical implications of the use of research to guide health education program planning in general? For national-level planning in developing countries?

10. What kind of compensations can be provided to couples who feel (and may be right) that at least three or more children are needed to provide for family support in the parents' old age?

#2 — SIZING UP THE NEWSPAPERS

Summary • Background • Results •
Commentary • Suggestions for Discussion

SUMMARY

On Saturday, June 29, 1974, a quarter-page ad appeared in five newspapers in Taiwan at a cost of approximately US$2,500. A return coupon offered a contraceptive sample or educational materials free. 11,530 persons requested these. The ad cost per person returning the coupon was US23¢. The cost per coupon returned ranged widely by newspaper: from US13¢ to US91¢. Nearly half the respondents were men, for whom the ongoing program had few services at all.

BACKGROUND

Previous Newspaper Usage

The family planning program in Taiwan has been using the newspaper on a limited basis in the following ways:

1. news releases on national and international activities and new developments in contraception;
2. articles and question and answer columns on methods and dealing with side-effects, on family and women's pages;
3. essay contests on contraceptive experience, advantages of small family, critiques of family planning TV programs; and
4. interviews of government officials, county/city councilmen on topics related to family planning.

Little of this was paid for by the family planning program.

Political, Budgetary and Educational Considerations

As indicated earlier, use of the mass media was a long time coming in the Taiwan family planning program. One major reason, of course, was the program's long-time "unofficial" status. Even after the program had been officially and publicly sanctioned by the Government in mid-1968, it took quite some while to overcome bureaucratic resistance to change. And even more time for the research and evaluation unit to recognize the need to gather information on the composition of the audience for mass media. By the 1970's, mass media audience survey modules had been integrated into the annual and bi-annual KAP (Knowledge, Attitude and Practice and Fertility) surveys begun in the early 1960's. These large-scale (several thousand respondents) stratified random sample surveys have been a major source of information for fertility trends and program guidelines. In spite of the considerable data available on media use and some perceptive analysis of listeners/readers/viewers, relatively little experimental study had been done on the effect of the media.

Furthermore, newspapers had received less attention than would seem desirable. Most of what coverage there was was free and generated partially by the health education unit of the family planning program.

One constraint concerning the previous use of the newspaper had been budgetary. Funds were not sufficient to implement an overall mass media program. Cost-effectiveness was a major consideration. Another constraint was political. As the program expanded in the 1970's, as well as its budget, the possibility of purchasing a space of the program's own choice in a paper of its own choice became feasible. At the same time, however, there persisted a throwback from the previous "informal" program when publicity in the media was sometimes best avoided for sound political reasons. There was considerable concern expressed by program staff that choosing one newspaper to buy advertising space from might cause hard feelings at another. Past experience provided testimony that blowing up minor happenings to major incidents was not uncommon among newsmen. Indeed, newspaper reporting of public health events had helped to shorten the careers of several public health leaders. There also was the less subtle dilemna that staff at governmental agencies were under the impression that ads must be placed in governmental newspapers. Part of this thinking may have been mistaken allegiance to other governmental agencies. On the other hand, some of it was gratitude for the governmental newspaper had backed the program in many subtle as well as obvious ways during its "unofficial" days. There also was the simple constraint that few real Island-wide audience surveys existed and circulation figures provided by newspapers were viewed with considerable skepticism by the observant individual, business or agency.

Another major constraint was an educational approach which traditionally tended to view the woman as the initiator of contraception rather than the male (prompted partly by budgetary constraints). One barrier still prevalent is the reluctance to reach the important younger and unmarried generation (or cohort for the demographers), primarily for reasons related to culture and morality. Adolescent pregnancy has become a serious problem, largely being ignored.

Purpose and Plan

It was in this historical context that this simple study of the effect and cost-effectiveness of a mass medium was implemented. In order to test the cost-

Name _____ Sex _____ Education _____				

Name _____ Sex _____ Education _____

Address _____

Single _____ Newly-Wed _____ Married _____

Number of Children: None _____ Boy _____ Girl _____

Contraceptive Experience: Yes ___ No ___ Using Now _____

Sample Requested (Limited to One)

   Loop Coupon _____ Pill Coupon (one cycle)_____

   Condom (half dz.) _____ Rhythm Calculator _____

Reading Material Requested (Limited to One)

   Handbook for Youth _____ For Newly-Wed _____ For Married_____

   Happy Family _____ Summer Night Dream_____ Late Happiness _____

Figure 4. Newspaper ad coupon.

effectiveness of a newspaper ad, to compare cost-effectiveness among different papers, and also to publicize the "Taichung Spacing Incentive Project" (see Appendix D), a quarter-page ad was placed in five leading newspapers in Taiwan: three Island-wide (*United Press, Central Daily News,* and *China Times*) and two regional (*Taiwan Daily News* in Central Taiwan (Taichung area) and *Taiwan Times* in the south).

For purposes of comparison, the same size ad (same content) was placed on the same day on the same page of all papers (back page, except *Taiwan Daily News,* which was on the first page because the back page was sold out).

The ad, in two colors, consisted of a picture of bride and groom, family planning guidance, a mail-in coupon, and announcement of the Taichung Spacing Incentive Project.

The coupon could be clipped out to send in (with return postage enclosed) to request one kind of contraceptive sample and one family planning educational booklet (see Figure 4). The coupon would contain information on the respondents' vital characteristics and previous contraceptive experience.

RESULTS

By July 16 (cut-off date), there were 11,530 newspaper coupons returned. Return postage had to be sent with the coupon, due to a limited project budget. About half came in the first two days. The total advertising fee was NT$101,350, which means a per case cost of NT$8.8 for the five papers used (exclusive of samples and materials sent, which were partially covered by the excess stamps enclosed for return postage). The cost for the *United Press* was the lowest (NT$5.02). The *Taiwan Times* was the highest (NT$34.64). It is worth noting that two Island-wide papers, the *United Press* and *China Times* got 3.6 times as many responses as the third, the *Central Daily News* (the government paper) for less than twice the total cost. Furthermore, the two regional papers cost NT$35 and NT$33 (per coupon returned) vs. the NT$5, NT$6, and NT$11 of the Island-wide papers (see Table 2).

Interestingly, more than 60 per cent of the requests were for rhythm method calculators (7,333 of 11,530); 2,607 requested condoms; 511 oral contraceptive coupons; and 456 Loop (IUD) coupons. Since there were only 620 rhythm calculators available, priority was given to married women with senior high and above education (who were thought to be able to better use these). Married men with lower education were given condoms (sent to 3,000 persons, six condoms per person). Women received a free cycle of pills at the health station. Unmarried persons were given educational materials. It should be noted that 48 per cent of respondents were males. This seems compatible with the larger male readership of newspapers revealed in some surveys. This strong interest and the tendency of the program to be female-centered in both educational approaches and service reinforced the need for program review of this matter.

Vital data for the 11,530 were put on IBM cards and analyzed in terms of age, sex, marital status, parity, residence, education, and previous contraceptive experience. Individual newspapers were reviewed in terms of "reader profiles" to help education staff better plan materials for them. It was found in later follow-up that half of all loop and pill coupons sent to respondents were used. The project was funded by a grant from the Population Council as part of a larger project to try out ways to reach younger couples.

Table 2. Comparative Costs Per Respondent Per Newspaper

Newspapers	United Press	China Times	Central Daily News	Taiwan Daily News	Taiwan Times
Number of Respondents	4,658 (40%)	3,636 (31.5%)	2,284 (19.8%)	480 (4.2%)	394 (3.4%)
Ad Cost (NT$)	23,400	23,400	25,000	15,900	13,650
Cost Per Respondents (NT$)[a]	5.02	6.44	10.95	33.13	34.64

[a] NT$1 = US2.5¢.

COMMENTARY

An interesting interaction of budgetary, cultural and program factors continued to restrain the Taiwan family planning program in its efforts to reach younger persons (both in the school setting as well as through the mass media) and males. More is said about this elsewhere in this book. Political and bureaucratic/organizational considerations also intertwine with these factors in the case of the use of newspapers for public education purposes.

In retrospect, this study clearly indicated that certain newspapers are probably more cost-effective than others although probably most staff engaged in the program administration already knew it. It, however, was one thing to know fewer people read the Government paper, and another to be able to demonstrate the study findings to administrators in charge of budgets.

The advantage of this study was its cost-effectiveness feedback component: the focus on the clear-cut advantages from an educational and service provision of selecting the appropriate paper, i.e., the number of persons taking action recommended per unit of cost. Little difference in terms of socio-demographic variables was found among the newspaper audiences. All seemed to be reaching similar audiences. Obviously, it was not possible to measure political orientations of the audience nor of the credibility of private versus governmental newspapers or national versus regional. The extent to which the public *trusts* or believes there is *expertise* in a particular newspaper seems important. Or again, the public trust in the source of the information in the ad, i.e., the Taiwan Family Planning Program. Generally speaking, we know more about audience, message, channel and effects than source.

Another relevant factor in the implementation of this project was that it was part of an in-service training seminar held bi-weekly for staff of the research and evaluation and also the health education program divisions of the Institute of Family Planning. Through this seminar, staff of the research and the program units worked together to plan, implement, and actually evaluate this newspaper study and to apply the findings to their other programmatic efforts. It, of course, was possible to conduct this experiment and to have it funded as part of a larger project designed to provide incentives to younger married women to space between children and postpone a first birth (The Taichung Spacing Incentive Project) which is described in Appendix D. In effect, an experiment was piggybacked within an experiment and the results were disseminated not only to Taiwan but to the other countries involved in the funding of the project (funded through the International Committee on Applied Research in Population) as a demonstration which would be of interest to them (in this case, South Korea, Bangladesh, Indonesia, Philippines, and Thailand).

SUGGESTIONS FOR DISCUSSION

1. Imagine that you are the Director of the family planning program described here. You have just listened to a presentation by the Chief of Research and Evaluation of the results of the study described here. What are the recommendations for program action you would expect to hear? Which ones would you not expect to be given to you? Why? Which recommendations are you likely to implement? Why?

2. Imagine that you are the Chief of the Research and Evaluation Division. Prepare a brief memo listing the major study results and your recommendations for action. Which would you expect to see action on? Why do you think the Director will act or not act?

3. Select two persons to take on the roles above. Ask the Research and Evaluation Chief to prepare the memo. Ask the Director to write down beforehand what he expects the Chief to recommend for action. Compare the two: the Director's expectation and the R & E Chief's actual recommendations. Ask the audience beforehand to list how the two will agree or differ and why.

4. Imagine you are a member of the Education Evaluation Seminar mentioned in this case. You are planning this study and have listed several hypotheses you would like to explore. These are: 1) that a certain paper will reach younger males; 2) that certain content in articles will reach adolescents; 3) that certain papers will reach lower socio-economic groups; and 4) that people trust one paper more than another. To what extent do you think that the other staff in your agency already think they have the answers to these questions. If they have the answers, why bother researching these topics? What is the relevance of the "researcher's dilemma?" (See Chapter 2.)

#3 — HOW NOT TO PRICE ORAL CONTRACEPTIVES

Summary • Tale of Three Townships • Results • Commentary • Suggestions for Discussion

SUMMARY

This case study shows clearly that research findings did not always find their way into program use. It also illustrates two of the many reasons which hinder application of research results:

1. lack of available funds to implement findings; and
2. time lag (by the time findings were available for program use, the program was ahead of the study).

TALE OF THREE TOWNSHIPS

It was not until January 1967 that oral contraceptives became available on an island-wide scale (and then only to those who had discontinued IUDs or had contraindications to IUD usage). To prepare for wider-scale use, a study was initiated in August 1966 to determine whether women would accept the pill, at what price the pill would be more acceptable, whether women would continue use, and what side effects or educational problems there might be.

The pills were offered for NT$10 (US25¢), NT$5 (US12.5¢), and free in three townships near the program headquarters in Taichung City. A previous small-scale test offered the pills by mail at NT$20 per cycle (the drugstore price was NT$40-50 per cycle). The townships were selected on the basis of matching for various criteria. In order to simulate what would be the likely situation in a program in which a variety of contraceptive methods would be offered, village health education nurses offered couples a choice of the pill, the Lippes loop, foam tablets, condoms, or sterilization. All methods were offered at reduced cost: NT$5 for a box of foam tablets, NT$5 for a dozen condoms, NT$300 (US$7.50) for tubal ligation, NT$200 (US$5) for vasectomy, pills at NT$10, $5, and free (depending on the townships). The village health education nurses (VHEN) were somewhat different from regular Pre-pregnancy Health (PPH) workers in that they were mobile workers who moved from village to village providing health education, sanitation, MCH, and family planning. PPH workers dealt with family planning only.

RESULTS

On November 15, 1967 (after fifteen months in two townships and fourteen months in the third), the study ended. The results indicated (see Table 3):

1. that there was not much difference between NT$5 and free but that in the NT$10 area, only about half as many new cases were recruited for the oral contraceptives;
2. that a fairly large percentage of acceptors could be recruited in a relatively short time (averaging 8.4 per cent of married women twenty to forty-four in fourteen to fifteen months); and
3. that continuation rates were low, as indicated by the usage index developed.

This last finding proved to have considerable significance for overall program expansion in Taiwan since women stopped use of the oral contraceptives quickly and overall continuation rates were among the lowest of all Asian programs. One factor affecting this low continuation undoubtedly was side effects but another was lack of field staff faith in the method. A later survey of staff in 1970 indicated that few fieldworkers used the pill and fewer still ever intended to use it.

During the study, Population Studies Center staff interviewed the field workers on many occasions. A follow-up survey of 128 acceptors also was carried out in September 1967 to find out who stopped pill use and why. In addition, a survey of 504 women who did not accept any methods, was carried out to determine if they had known about the pills and why they had not tried them.

Table 3. Three Township Pill Study (August 1966 to November 1967): Results

(1)	(2)	(3)	(4)	(5)	(6)	(7)
				Rate of		
Township (Cost)	No. of Wives 20-44	Total No. Pill Acceptors	Total No. Cycles Distributed	Acceptance Per Cent (3)/(2)	Cumul. Month Observation	Usage Index[a] (4)/(6)
Ta-an (NT$10)	2,558	146	227	5.7%	1,828	12.4%
Hsien-Hsi (NT$5)	1,726	177	345	10.3%	1,212	28.5%
Ta-tu (Free)	3,332	316	400	9.5%	1,684	23.8%
TOTAL	7,616	639	972	8.4%	4,724	20.6%

SOURCE: Cernada and Sun, *East-West Communication Institute Papers*, No. 10, p. 26, 1974.

[a] An indicator used by the Taiwan Population Studies Center to show the "density" of use of pill cases.

Interestingly, although the results indicated that NT$10 produced far fewer acceptors, the island-wide oral contraceptive program which began in late January 1967 started providing the pill for NT$10 per cycle. This was in spite of the findings that a "contribution" of NT$5 produced an acceptance rate about double that of NT$10 and about the same rate as if the pills were offered free. One major reason why the research findings were not put into operation was largely that program administrators had a limited supply of pills (donated by the Population Council from Searle on a one-time basis) and they needed funds quickly so that they could start a revolving fund to purchase more supplies. This decision was made by the three key Committee members who were the policy-makers at that time (before an official policy supporting the family planning program existed).

COMMENTARY

In summary, the study's "operational validity" may be questioned (at least in retrospect) since the study results could not have been applied given the budget. The fact, however, was that at the time the study began, nobody knew what the cost of the orals to the program was going to be, nor that a revolving fund was possible under existing regulations regarding use of outside assistance. Local ingenuity concocted a "contribution" rather than a fee system and a quasi-voluntary agency was used to receive the funds.

The decision on price was not easy. Cost estimates ranged as high as 15 to 20 US cents (NT$6-8) per cycle for a small order. The NT$10 (US25¢) figure was chosen to provide the minimum amount needed for a revolving fund to purchase a continued supply for an estimated 20,000 users when the free 250,000 cycles ran out. The price of NT$20 (US50¢) in the mailing study had seemed too high; only 42 per cent had continued use in Taichung City after twelve months. Later continuation rates elsewhere proved even lower.

By the end of 1967, a price of NT$4-5 per cycle (US10.8¢) was negotiated (on the basis of the Swedish International Development Agency wholesale purchase prices) and 200,000 cycles purchased. By late 1968, another inter-national donor had agreed to provide pill supplies free, and in May of 1970, the "service fee" for pills dropped from NT$10 to NT$1. At that time, monthly numbers of new pill acceptors more than doubled from the 2,500 level to nearly 6,000.

It is doubtful that decisionmakers could have been convinced to set the pill prices at lower than NT$10, considering the financial problem involved. Furthermore, even had they been convinced, the study was too late to affect the action program decision. It took time to gather results and the program was moving too rapidly to wait. Decisions had to be made and budgetary figures were the first available to be considered. Possibly the study might have been started earlier than August 1966; but there was no indication until early 1966 that the pills might be available at an affordable wholesale price. The study might have shown results more clearly had there been more emphasis on the pill and less on the cafeteria of other methods offered (IUD, foam tablets, male and female sterilization). In any case it seems that price made a difference, judging by the spurt in monthly acceptances once the price was reduced — although perhaps the fixing of the higher price followed by a "bargain" lower price helped also in this respect.

In a sense, in concentrating attention on getting the pills into the program so that people had more choices of contraceptives, the program paid less attention to the attitude of the workers and the public to the method. This is not to say that researchers and program personnel were not aware of the problems but that their possible significance in a larger-scale program expansion was less apparent at the time.

SUGGESTIONS FOR DISCUSSION

1. One assumption made by the Taiwan planners seems to have been that supplies should not be offered free. To what extent was this assumption based on program needs? Are items offered at no cost less desirable? How would a sliding scale fee have fit into this program? What might have been the effect of supervising such a scale in the field?

2. If you were the program administrator, what would you (with benefit of hindsight) have done to help eliminate the "timing" problem in this study? Do you know of other program situations where timing gaps have occurred in applied research?

3. When this family planning program began, oral contraceptives cost so much that they were ruled out of the program. Furthermore, in Taiwan the intrauterine contraceptive had a long-time history of popularity. The intent of offering the oral contraceptive was to provide people in Taiwan with more contraceptive choice. To what extent do you think people in the country should be involved in such a decision? In what ways could this be done?

4. One major drawback to this study may have been that the fieldworkers themselves had little interest in using this contraceptive. Later studies showed some antipathy to the pill among fieldworkers. To what extent do programs you know of measure staff knowledge, perceptions, attitude and practices regarding the services they provide?

#4 — PASTING YOUR UMBRELLA BEFORE THE RAIN*

Summary • Identifying the Need • Deciding to Do It and Getting the Money • Doing the Job • Interpreting the Research • Commentary • Suggestions for Discussion

SUMMARY

This case study tells how the results of large-scale social surveys and demographic projections are translated into educational program objectives and, more importantly, an educational product that gears into the thinking patterns of a younger generation. Cultural, bureaucratic and political obstacles to change and how they were overcome are reviewed in this chronological unfolding of the development of Taiwan's first population education approach in the classroom.

The process about to be described took about a year and a half. The result was a forty-five page supplementary text distributed to all 400,000 graduating junior high, senior high, and vocational school students throughout Taiwan in April 1971. In candor, it should be said that it took a year and a half to finish this job not only due to the careful planning and integration of study findings into the text or to the pretesting among those students for whom it was intended, or to the evaluation of changes in knowledge and attitude levels among students purportedly induced by the text. The major reason for the long period of time taken to produce the slender volume discussed in this case study was quite uncomplicated. As stated in the English translation of the text which was printed for distribution abroad, the major problem was that "it was the first time such a publication had been attempted in Taiwan . . . and nearly everybody who would have any responsibility was afraid of getting into trouble." [45]

Such fears were understandable. Precedents were hard to come by. Although there were many active family planning programs throughout the world by 1969 when this project began (perhaps forty national programs covering about 70 per cent of the population of developing countries), those using the school systems to help curb population growth were few indeed. Although western scholarly journals exhibited a great deal of interest in the subject and it had many proponents, particularly among American educators involved in (or hoping to launch a mid-career transition to) the international circuit, relatively little in the way of production or distribution of such educational materials had taken place in the developing countries. Considering that public health agencies and teacher training institutions had a good deal of experience in developing curricula,

*The author is grateful for suggestions made by J. F. Tsai, L. C. Niu, L. P. Lu, O. D. Finnigan, C. C. Cernada, and S. M. Keeny.

teacher training and teaching materials for integrating communicable disease and health and hygiene preventive concepts into Taiwan's schools, the absence in the population area is notable.

The colorfully illustrated booklet, "Paste Your Umbrella Before the Rain," which ultimately was produced, contained information on world population trends, their consequences for Taiwan as a whole and for the individual living there. Its major focus, however, was on the supposed interests of graduating students: the importance to the individual of going on to higher education to get a better job, of later marriage, of postponing having children, having fewer of them and caring for them well, and spacing between births. Taking control of one's future by careful planning of one's total life was stressed. (See Figure 5.)

It took Taiwan a relatively long time to come to the realization that the birth rates would not just keep on dropping as they had over the previous recent years.

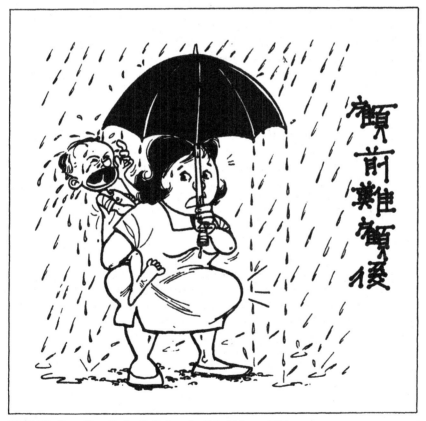

SOURCE: *Paste Your Umbrella Before the Rain*, Taiwan, 1971.

Figure 5. Not easy to care for both.

It was not enough to expend all the program's staff time and funds on an audience of only married couples. Sometime, about 1967, the program "woke up with a shock" as the author of the English edition of the booklet pointed out in the Preface. "Because of a baby boom in the early 1950's, the percentage of marriageable young women in 1972 was going to be 60 per cent more than in 1968. They would be highly fertile and, by Chinese custom, would mostly have babies before they had been married a year." [1] Program analysis of ongoing research also had begun to show by 1968 that the organized family planning program had had little effect on the younger married women (e.g., ages twenty-five to twenty-nine) and, indeed, that the fertility of the married women less than twenty-five years old had risen over the past decade. And in spite of the efforts of the program, the so-called preferred number of children a married woman wanted had dropped in five years only from 4 to 3.8, with a preference for two sons. It only seemed logical on the basis of research findings for the family planning program to review its audiences and to determine how best to meet needs and consider creating demand for services by more and varied educational inputs. High school students were easily identified as a potential audience for the proposed educational approaches. As logical a target group as they seemed in terms of applied research findings, however, reaching them turned out to be an immense and elaborate undertaking as our case study will illustrate.

IDENTIFYING THE NEED

The Chinese have a saying that "a thousand mile journey begins with a single step." This is the story of how Taiwan took that first step toward reaching young, unmarried students and helping them become more aware of the advantages of a planned, smaller family.

1959-1961

In 1959, the Governor of Taiwan agreed to set up pre-pregnancy health (PPH) services at local government health stations. By 1963, 120 of the 361 local health stations had added full time PPH workers to offer family planning services through home visiting. In 1961, the Taiwan Population Studies Center was established as a research unit. It later became responsible for both research and action programs as the Family Planning Institute (FPI) under the auspices of the Taiwan Provincial Health Department.

1961-Early 1968

The present family planning service program started from the PPH service program at local health stations and the classic Taichung City experiment in 1962 which was extended island-wide in 1964. As the program developed, it became increasingly obvious to program implementors and Provincial Public Health administrators that, even with a staff of 360 lay workers to recruit clients, provision of contraceptive services alone could not do the job of reducing the population growth rate from 3 per cent to 2 per cent by the end of 1973, and sustain this reduction. Other sectors had to cooperate to help spread the word about services and, more importantly, to begin challenging traditional ideas about completed family size. A Population Policy Study Committee of the Ministry of the Interior worked from 1964 to 1966 on a set of regulations governing the implementation of family planning and an outline of population policy. When these regulations were officially adopted, in May 1968, the population problem began to emerge from the health services, and become more of an obvious national problem, calling for cooperation from many agencies for solution.

From early 1968, members of the Taiwan Provincial Family Planning Institute, resident foreign advisors of the Population Council (a U.S. based international educational foundation) and the UNICEF Representative had been discussing ways in which family planning could be supported by agencies other than health. One approach could be through the School Health Committee of the Ministry of Education (MOE). In fact, Dr. S. P. Lee then Chairman of the Health Education Department of National Taiwan Normal University did manage to obtain MOE approval for two chapters on family life and reproductive physiology, both of which appeared in junior high school health texts starting in 1968. No attempt, however, was made to produce a separate text on population and family planning, or to integrate these materials into other subjects, due to lack of guidelines from the National Government defining the support required from the Ministry of Education at the National level, the Taiwan Education Department (PED) at the Provincial level and the Taipei Bureau of Education, at the Taipei City level.

Mid-1968

The Population Council resident education advisor was requested by the Taiwan Provincial Institute of Family Planning to collect available materials on population education in India and Pakistan where he was scheduled to consult. He did so and also visited with faculty at Teachers College, Columbia University, to review progress in population education to date. The clearest finding was that there were few materials adaptable to Taiwan and that most of the literature consisted of academic discussion of the pros and cons of various approaches.

Late 1968

UNICEF agreed to provide vehicles and motorcycles for the Taiwan family planning program as the United Nations policy toward family planning became more favorable and local support clearer. To date, the U.N., particularly WHO, had ducked the issue in Taiwan.

April 1969

The National Government announced an official national policy supporting the control of population growth. This announcement theoretically opened the door for broadening the family planning education approach beyond home visiting and mass media to the school system.

May-July 1969

In early May, visiting University of Michigan Population Studies Center researchers helped pinpoint more clearly the extent of the increasing numbers of younger women in Taiwan. By 1972, the number of women ages twenty to twenty-four would increase by 60 per cent over 1968's number (from 460,000 to 750,000). If their age-specific fertility rates remained the same, Taiwan's birth rate would soar.

This reason for reaching young women was tied in with a list of suggestions for program actions to be taken by all public agencies, prepared by the Family Planning Institute (FPI) and Population Council staff and submitted to then Minister of Finance, K. T. Li. The list indicated the need to integrate "population education into the regular curriculum of the secondary schools." This list contained suggestions for the broad spectrum of agencies in government to begin to help curb population growth.

The logical approach would have been to get the National Ministry of Education involved in providing a population textbook. The problem was that to get a textbook cleared would take years. Revisions of the textbook system are on certain schedules, and go through intensive and long-time screening. Furthermore, the Ministry of Education is often being petitioned by various groups to introduce textbooks on other matters. Their official view as presented on several occasions was that they were already overworked. "If population is added, then traffic safety, tax collection, etc., will have to be added for other government agencies." Accordingly, it was decided to try a "supplementary" text, which would come under the auspices of the Taiwan Provincial Education department. An outline of a population education booklet with an estimated budget was prepared and discussed with the local UNICEF representative in Taipei. An informal request was made to him for US$25,000 (equivalent NT$) for printing a booklet on the value of having a small family, to be used as supplementary teaching material or as part of a regular course in the high schools. The submission of this request was preceded by several meetings with the UNICEF representative wherein it was decided that the booklet was in line with UNICEF's function, and a tangible project which was more likely to get UNICEF funding than were vague discussions of ways to integrate teaching into the school curriculum. It also was a routine project as a supplementary booklet and the decision to approve it was within the discretion of the local UNICEF representative's powers (subject to approval at Bangkok Regional Headquarters). Perhaps, as importantly, the Government was behind in its production of supplementary texts under UNESCO technical guidance and UNICEF subsidy of paper and ink for printing. A booklet of this sort would make up for as many as eight booklets in the UNESCO series. Furthermore, there was pressure applied by the former UNICEF Regional Representative who now served a similar regional role with the Population Council, advising family planning programs in East Asia. The UNICEF representative was agreeable and enthusiastic; and the Family Planning Institute and Population Council staff committed themselves to doing the job of writing and editing the proposed booklet.

September 1969

The first meeting of the inter-agency committee to implement the suggestions to involve all government agencies was called at the National level by the Population Division of the Ministry of Interior and held in the National Capital, Taipei. In addition to the Education Ministry, there were staff attending from the Ministry of Interior, the Council for International Economic Cooperation and Development (CIECD), the Executive Yuan, the National Defense Ministry, the Ministry of Communications, the Ministry of Finance, the Provincial Health Department, the Taipei City Health Bureau, and the Taiwan Family Planning Institute. It was clear from the tone of the meeting that the related agencies were expected to take some action. The list of suggestions mentioned earlier was presented by Finance Minister K. T. Li and discussed and screened for feasibility. Conclusions were issued calling for increased cooperation from various National government agencies, the Province of Taiwan and Taipei City. It was made clear that at both National and Provincial levels, Education officials were expected to cooperate. Family Planning Institute staff brought these instructions to the attention of officials of the Taiwan Provincial Education Department who were responsible for reviewing and publishing text books for all schools in the Province of Taiwan.

DECIDING TO DO IT AND GETTING THE MONEY

Not all such interagency meetings bring immediate results. Coordination is a major problem and not easily achieved. Follow-up often is ignored. This one was an exception as the calendar of events which follows demonstrates.

October 1969

The Health Commissioner agreed to do the booklet on the advantages of the small family with the proviso that:

1. UNICEF would fund;
2. the Government policy was favorable; and
3. the Population Council would do an English language outline in consultation with Family Planning Institute personnel.

He also agreed to call on the Provincial Commissioner of Education to get his agreement to approve the use of the booklet in the schools.

November 1969

UNICEF felt that it was essential to have UNESCO backing in this project since UNESCO's official function was to provide technical inputs into the formal education system. The result was an agreement that UNICEF was to fund the booklet as proposed, and that UNESCO would be involved in any longer-term planning for the school curriculum. Their full agreement was conveyed to the Provincial Education Department officials with a request that planning begin.

DOING THE JOB

December 1969/January 1970

Procedure — Family Planning Institute and Population Council personnel met with Taiwan Provincial Education Department officials informally over tea and obtained the Provincial Education Department's preliminary agreement to what the outline of such a booklet might be if it were to be considered for use in Taiwan. It was explained that, due to lack of funds, the booklet might have to be provided only to female students. It was informally agreed that, functionally, the Population Council advisor would help coordinate the project among the various agencies since nobody else had authority to move among agencies at various Governmental agencies. Also he and his staff were to help with an initial booklet outline in English which would take advantage of work done elsewhere which might fit Taiwan's particular cultural setting. The Family Planning Institute would rewrite and modify the booklet in Chinese; and the Provincial Education Department would adapt it to the high school level.

Choice of Method — It became clear at this point that the booklet was more acceptable than any other approach since it would not have to go through "formal" clearance with the National-level Ministry of Education in Taipei as the booklet would not be officially "required" in the standard curriculum. Such clearance was estimated to take at least two years. There also was little evidence of interest in working on population education activities at the Ministry.

Content — It also became clear after the second meeting that the key decision-maker was the Executive Secretary of the Provincial Education Department and that he felt that Sex Education or mention of contraceptives was *NOT* suitable for high school students. Furthermore, he did not want to produce a booklet which was too "western" in its approach. The Commissioner of Education, however, had agreed to do the project, as he indicated, and he would try to adapt the draft prepared by the Institute and "foreign" advisor. After meeting with the Executive Secretary, the booklet was discussed in greater detail with the Chief of the Provincial Education Department's School Health Committee (which linked public health and school health activities and had produced booklets in cooperation with UNICEF before) under whose jurisdiction the project fell.

The lesson learned from these preliminary sessions was that the Provincial Education Department's Executive Secretary wanted reassurance of the Government's firm backing and that there would be no unnecessary foreign influence. The Family Planning Institute provided him with the September 1969 recommendations of the Executive Yuan that more Government agencies, including Education, become involved in population activities. It also provided reassurance as to the good intentions and technical expertise of the Population Council advisor. He was known to be neither an advocate of sex education nor a subversive — and acting at the request of the Government.

February/March 1970

The population education approach adopted for the draft booklet included: a basic introduction to population dynamics; a basic understanding of human reproduction; an understanding of health problems associated with childbearing; an appreciation of the relationship between quality of life for a family and family size; an appreciation of the significance of population growth for social and economic development; a familiarity with the population problem in Taiwan. The first rough draft was prepared in English by Population Council staff.

April 1970

Funding possibilities now that material was real were increasing. It was decided to try to provide the booklet to all graduating high school, junior high and junior college students, including both males and females. To do so, 400,000 copies would be needed in 1971. The UNICEF contribution was therefore matched by funds from the Family Planning Institute. It was decided to concentrate mainly on the small family ideal, and to tie this in with development and rising standard of life for the family. A primary resource was a booklet prepared first in 1963 and revised in 1968 which was used to train field workers to talk with women. This booklet spoke very simply of planning for the future, the health of mothers and children, and family economics.

The first English draft was reviewed by twelve health educators from the Family Planning Institute and the Taiwan Provincial Health Department who suggested that the material be reorganized, factual references be added, local examples be amplified and the text be made more consistent with Taiwanese culture. The emphasis remained on the concept of planning — to get more education, to get a better job, to marry only when ready, and to plan for a desired number of children.

June/July 1970

A quick translation of the draft booklet was prepared and pretested with twenty-four teachers and eighty students. Reactions were generally favorable but it seemed that there ought to be more emphasis on jobs and family responsibilities for those not planning to attend college. There also needed to be more pictures and practical examples.

A meeting of UNICEF, PED, PHD, and PC officials was held to get approval to proceed and to settle the question of funding and sponsorship. It was determined that the Family Planning Institute would cover the cost of writing, printing, and delivery; that UNICEF would provide paper and ink; that PED would provide a mailing list of schools and specify the number of copies required to be sent; and that PHD would act as publisher. The PED Executive Secretary was pleased to see the Chinese version and that the pretest had indicated reader interest and no backlash. It was agreed that a professional writer should be hired to simplify the Chinese and to rewrite the book so that it would be more in line with government education policy which was to encourage technical and vocational training. Also, items such as the "advantage of working and postponing marriage to build up a dowry" were to be excluded since they were against official government policy — however, realistic they might be.

One of the serious disadvantages to the option of producing a supplementary booklet was that the contents would not be questioned in the standard curriculum exams. In a system which implicitly, if not explicitly, stresses rote learning and feedback of school text materials and teacher lectures, a "supplemental" item often is ignored. In other words, if it was not required reading and in the exam, it probably would not be read.

The question was "How to be sure students read the book?" The answer was that the FPI could provide funds for a national essay contest to promote its reading. In addition, a Teacher's Guide was developed to help the teachers use the materials.

At a subsequent working meeting, the length of the text, the number of pictures, the inclusion of charts, the size of the book, the schedule for writing and printing, and an estimated budget were worked out.

August 1970

The professionally written draft was produced and sent to the PED and FPI for review.

September 1970

A second pretest among eighteen teachers and sixty students was held and the results obtained and analyzed by October 1. A dozen cartoon pictures were produced to be integrated into the text to liven up the pictorial presentation (see Figure 6).

October 1970

A meeting of PC, UNICEF, PED, PHD, and the writer was held to secure final approval of the draft text and the pictorial material. Because of pre-test comments by students and teachers it was decided to include information as to

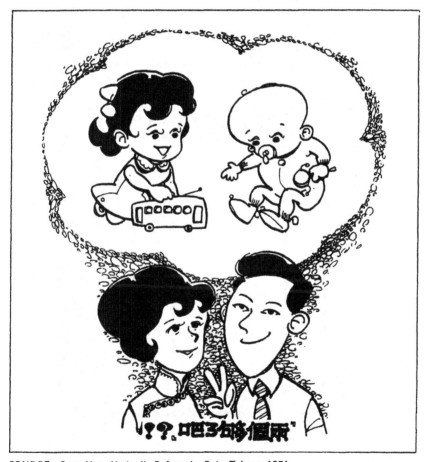

SOURCE: *Paste Your Umbrella Before the Rain*, Taiwan, 1971.

Figure 6. Two are enough?

the location of family planning services in the community as a final note in the text. PED was satisfied with this version and turned the project over to PHD, the FPI, and UNICEF.

November 1970

Minor revisions of the drawings were made, a population pyramid and a growth curve were added, and the book was sent through UNICEF to the printer. (See Figure 7.) An English retranslation also was completed to distribute abroad to educational leaders who had been thinking about doing something like this but had not gotten started as yet.

December 1970

The first page proofs were received from the printer and minor revisions were made. Copies of the English version were mailed to overseas consultants for comment (and, of course, to let others know that Taiwan preferred to do more than talk about the subject as most other countries were confined to doing to date).

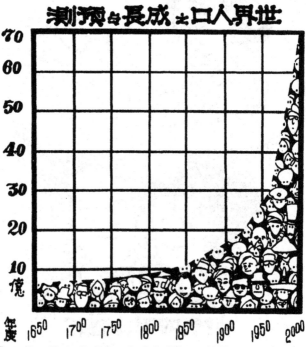

SOURCE: *Paste Your Umbrella Before the Rain*, Taiwan, 1971.
NOTE: Numbers of people are measured by "Yi" or 100,000,000. Ten yi equals one billion.

Figure 7. Projection of world population growth.

Early 1971

The booklets were printed and shipped out on schedule via a commercial forwarding company which attended to the shipping for a cost of about $2,500. The plan of distribution was carefully worked out and the Taiwan Provincial Education Department supplied a list of schools and the number of copies to be sent to each. The Department also sent out a letter to each school with detailed instructions about distribution to be certain that the books would not remain unused in the school storage rooms.

The final cost was about U.S.7¢ per copy, including the cost of paper, ink, printing, text preparation, distribution, and contest prizes.

From an ancient Chinese proverb of unknown origin, came the booklet's title: "Paste Your Umbrella Before the Rain." One must always be prepared for what will happen next.

Spring 1971

What *we* were not prepared for was an error discovered on a single table in the booklet which appeared to indicate that Taiwan was a country (with which the Republic of China's National Government certainly does not agree). The Chinese National Security Administration (if its title can be so translated) insisted that the table had to be corrected. A similar error also was noted in the Teacher's Guide. All 400,000 books had to be collected from schools around the island, corrected, and then redistributed – at no small cost.

INTERPRETING THE RESEARCH

April 1971

The revised booklets were out in the schools – finally. To get this to happen again the next year, there had to be positive findings that the booklet made a difference at least in awareness and knowledge and, hopefully, attitude among the students. The Teacher's Guide already was not proving successful. Its orientation was too directed to providing more information on population demographic considerations: population and age structure, urbanization growth rates, population doubling time, dependency burden, density and policies. The problem was that it did not serve as a guide to the teacher as to how to use the "Paste Your Umbrella Before the Rain" booklet.

Accordingly, a pre-survey of 1,277 students who were to receive the supplementary booklet, and who were selected from twelve representative schools, took place in February 1971. This survey was done before distribution of "Paste Your Umbrella Before the Rain."

Table 4. Pre- and Post-Survey of Ideal Number of Children and Sons

	Pre-Survey Readers (N = 1277)	Post-Survey Readers (N = 1277)	Post-Survey Non-Readers (N = 74)	Control Readers (N = 511)
Ideal Number of Children	3.1	2.8	3.1	2.8
Ideal Number of Sons	1.8	1.6	1.8	1.6

SOURCE: *Annual Report*, Taiwan Provincial Institute of Family Planning, p. 16, 1971.

May 1971

After distribution of the text, another survey was taken in May to determine the short-term impact on the students. The 1,277 students who were in the pre-survey were re-interviewed. In addition, 174 students who did not receive the booklet were interviewed (to separate the effect of the booklet) as were an additional 511 students who were not part of the pre-survey (to control for pre-survey exposure). Results of the pre- and post-survey questions dealing with ideal number of children indicated a slightly lower ideal number of children (2.8 versus 3.1) and of sons (1.6 versus 1.8) among students after reading the booklet (see Table 4). Knowledge about population problems was measured by a series of eleven true or false questions and there was some improvement, with ability to answer questions correctly rising from 76 to 82 per cent. Ranking of Government priorities among problems and programs also saw population growth move from sixth before the booklet to first afterwards. The percentage of students who ranked population first, second, or third in priority increased from 38 per cent before reading the text to 58 per cent after. There are, of course, difficulties in having adequate controls for all potentially influencing variables including the passage of time and the surveys themselves. Perhaps, more likely, there is the possibility of acquiesence in responses to what the students think that the surveyor wanted to know. Nevertheless, there was positive feedback and ample information collected for needed revisions in the booklet.

August 1971

The post-survey conducted in late May was reported in early August to the appropriate governmental agency staff. The various agencies agreed to fund the booklet again. It has continued to be revised and re-issued now for more than a half-dozen editions and several million students even though the Population Council and UNICEF have long departed, the latter due to political changes at the United Nations and the former perhaps more due to its assessment that its advisory services were needed more elsewhere.

COMMENTARY

1. Synthesizing a variety of research findings into educational objectives for a printed booklet and still making it practically useful as well as interesting to the reader requires a skilled writer and editor as well as an audience survey to determine existing needs. This project was weakest in respect to knowing about its audience.

2. Pretesting the early draft booklet made a major difference in alerting writers and planners to what ought to be said and how to say it. Potential audiences need to be involved in all stages of preparation of educational materials and fact-finding studies.

3. Ethnocentricity plays a major role as an obstacle to social change and foreign assistance must maintain a low profile when it becomes involved in linkage among agencies or between research and applied program action.

4. Establishing linkages between agencies at different Governmental levels is essential if research findings are to be translated into program action. Bureaucracy demands that each unit give its stamp of approval and a "linker" is needed at each stage to guide the program through the maze.

5. Cultural, bureaucratic, and political obstacles to getting applied research findings into action existed. No one of these could be dealt with except in relation to others. Wherever innovative work is proposed such barriers will exist. One way to overcome some of these is through the *synergetic* effect of a well-coordinated group of forces continuing to try to bring about change. Another is having the results of the innovation (e.g., a pretest) on hand to demonstrate its quality and interest to its audience.

6. Moving beyond public health-centered family planning to other agencies is a difficult task. Not only do the other agencies have to see it as in their own best interest to act but public health sometimes has to learn to let go a little.

7. In retrospect, not enough was done to involve the National Ministry of Education in planning and this reflected itself in a lack of future action from this agency. The strongly ethnocentric views of this agency might have been capitalized on in some ways had there been more interaction in the booklet planning.

SUGGESTIONS FOR DISCUSSION

1. What kind of research do you think ought to be done on son preference? Why might there be difficulty in integrating findings into action programs?

2. What are the advantages to getting research applied of having a person involved in a project who can move freely among the various kinds and hierarchical levels of governmental agencies? What are the disadvantages?

3. What were the specific cultural barriers to implementation of this project? Bureaucratic barriers? Political barriers? What is similar about these three categories of barriers?

4. The Taiwan family planning program had a long-time history of disseminating results of its work to other countries. To what extent may this have influenced implementation of this project?

5. Getting population education out of the exclusive grasp of public health agencies and into other social action programs was a difficult task in Taiwan. To what extent are there similar problems in the United States in community health education? Do public health institutions sometimes hamper this branching out? Why?

6. "Population education" has had many connotations for administrators. It was vital to define just what the educational objectives of "Paste Your Umbrella Before the Rain" were and the content to carry these out. This specificity was needed for political reasons — to distinguish "population education" from "sex education" which had been linked with Communist movements. Are there similar backlash reactions to public health campaigns in the U.S.? Why? To what extent is it health education's fault?

#5 — FREE OFFERS FOR A LIMITED TIME ONLY

Summary • Reasons Why the Project Began • Results • Commentary • Suggestions for Discussion

SUMMARY

This is the story of an educational *gimmick*. Its history in marketing is ancient — the free offer for a limited time only. Its health educational theoretical basis lies in its trigger or cue to action. But it also served a secondary purpose in harnessing the creative enthusiasm of the field workers who seem to have put much more effort into their work during this "limited time" offering. The study illustrates:

1. the close attention the Taiwan program paid to feedback from both the consumers of service and the home-visiting family planning field worker; and

2. the flexibility of its applied research projects, particularly their continual and rapid adaptability to field problems.

REASONS WHY THE PROJECT BEGAN

During the early years of the Taiwan family planning program the mainstay of the staff was the "Pre-pregnancy Health" Worker, so-called euphemistically because of a lack of official Government policy supporting the family planning program. This worker was stationed at a rural township health station or an urban district station. She was usually married, had children, and was practicing contraception. She was trained for less than a month and then closely supervised in the field. Her major job was family planning. She copied the names of women who had three or more children from her township registration office and visited them at their home. Her job was to educate women about available ways to prevent conception and to help them get this service if they wanted it.

As part of her armamentarium, the PPH worker carried a block of coupons, one of which she would provide to a woman she visited who was interested in having an intrauterine contraceptive device. The coupon was a unique educational and evaluative method [38]. It was divided into three parts. Part 1 was kept by the worker as it provided the name and address of the coupon acceptor for follow-up purposes. Parts 2 and 3 were given to the woman who would bring them to a local private physician who had been contracted and trained by the family planning program. The coupon would entitle her to the IUD at half price. At the end of each month, someone from the County Health Bureau would visit the doctors and collect Part 2 of the coupons. The physician kept Part 3 of the coupon as a record of what she/he was to be paid (the family planning program subsidized half the IUD insertion price). The coupons (Part 2) then were reviewed in terms of job performance of each PPH worker by the County PPH Supervisor and then mailed to the program headquarters in Taichung where monthly characteristics of acceptors and results by each township were compiled and reported to the field. See Figure 8 for a sample of Part 2 of the coupon which was a mainstay of the ongoing program evaluation.

Most importantly, for purposes of our case study, the coupons offered the holder a 50 per cent discount on the cost of the IUD (the other half of the physician's payment being subsidized by the program).

Early experience with the IUD acceptor coupons in 1964 revealed that two to three times as many woman had accepted a coupon entitling them to IUD insertion at half price than had actually come to the clinics for IUD insertion. Many field workers expressed an interest in facilitating a woman's decision-making by having a limited time *free offer*. To find out if a free insertion with a specific time limit would bring in more acceptors, trial projects were conducted in two rural townships (population: 50,000) with low IUD acceptance rates. Field workers felt that a limited-time offer might be a stimulus to accept "*now* rather than later." Three months were believed to be long enough for the home visiting field worker to inform enough people about it, but short enough for action to be necessary soon. Workers were briefed and six of them distributed flyers to 8,080 households in six weeks. The flyers had information about contraceptives, where to get them and how to use them. Attached to it was the coupon, marked to indicate that "You can receive this contraceptive absolutely free if you go now before this special offer ends." The date of expiration was stamped on the coupon.

Earlier trial studies of six months' duration had not produced significant results — these were impressive! With the *free offer*, and limited time, 20 per cent, or 1,140, of the wives responded within three months and nearly two-thirds of these tried the IUD.

RESULTS

Administrators decided to see whether the success could be expanded on a larger scale. A *free offer* project was carried out from September to November 1965 in thirty townships where contraceptive acceptance was known to be low. There was a doubling of acceptors, and eventually some 180 townships (six groups of thirty each) received the treatment with equally good results.

THE COUPON USED FOR IUD PROGRAM

The following items will be filled out by the person who refers the case.

Name	Age
Name, Chief of Household	No. Living Children M ( ) F ( )
Address	
Name of Village	
Name of person referring case	
Type of person who referred PPH worker ( ) Practitioner ( ) VHEN ( ) Private Midwife ( ) Military Hospital ( ) Provincial Hospital ( ) Farmers' Association ( ) Health Bureau (Station) ( ) China Family Planning Association ( ) Others:	
Date of Issue:	

The following items will be filled out by the doctor who inserts the device.

Date of Insertion:
Type of Loop I (   )   II (   )   III (   )   IV (   )

Name of Clinic: Name of Doctor:

Address of Doctor:

Area Representative:

a) Do you want more children?

b) What was the contraceptive you last used?

c) When was your last childbirth?

(NT$30 will be paid by MCHA upon receipt of this coupon.)

SOURCE: Gillespie and Cernada, *Family Planning in Taiwan*, p. 132, 1966.

Figure 8. The coupon used for IUD program.

The effect of having free offers of IUD insertions for a period of three months in thirty selected townships may be seen from Figure 9. A look at the index for the three-month *free offer* period shows that there were at least twice as many insertions as during the preceding three-month period. These studies tried to demonstrate the effect of using such an offer to program administrators — especially the holders of the purse strings. Administrators, however, were skeptical. They noted that a drop usually occurred in the several months following the three-months *free offer.* Thereafter, the next test of free offers offered longer term observation. Data were included to show that although the acceptance rate lowered immediately following the free offer, it soon picked up again. As is clear, there is a decline following the three months after *free offer* period. This, however, was compensated for by a rise after the three month period (see Figure 9).

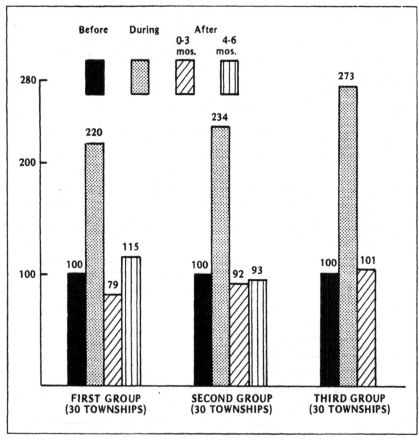

SOURCE: Taiwan Population Studies Center, *Taiwan's Family Planning in Charts,* 2nd edition, Taichung, 1967, p. 39.

Figure 9. Index of free insertions for a limited time only.

Eventually, the *free offer* program was expanded to include a mailing offer of a free IUD insertion to all recent postpartum women. It also was used on an island-wide basis during the last two weeks of 1966 and last twenty days of 1967 to help meet annual targets. This was essential in order to make use of funds budgeted which otherwise might be lost. This Island-wide basis caught on and was used thereafter for the last month or so of the budgetary year. Administrators who early were skeptical became convinced when they realized how quickly it enabled them to meet acceptor targets and to keep from losing unexpended funds.

COMMENTARY

Implications for research utilization drawn from this study include the following:

1. Whether the *"Free Offer* for a Limited Time Only" facilitated the public's decision-making or else the diffusion of information about the method (either through increased worker input and/or increased public diffusion by word-of-mouth) is not clear. It clearly, however, was effective in increasing acceptances of family planning methods.
2. The program started because the field workers recognized that people loved a bargain. Women had continued to ask them why they could not negotiate the price or have it at no cost. Field workers communicated their ideas on the potential value of this approach through the system of monthly meetings of field staff and quarterly meetings of field supervisors with headquarters evaluation and program staff. Local resident advisors also tried to serve as *linkers*, reinforcing the merits of this field worker suggestion to the program and evaluation staff and encouraging an action trial.
3. The suggestion fitted into the strong pattern of use of incentives developing in the program and which later blossomed into all sorts of field worker, acceptor, and even non-fertility incentives in Taiwan. And many other countries modeled themselves after Taiwan.
4. The excellent feedback system of service statistics through the coupon system enabled workers and headquarters to see the results rapidly — so that the program continued to expand to different areas and in different variations without any gap in reporting of results.
5. The pilot project gave the field worker the power to provide a bargain; enthused, she made as many as twice the usual number of home visits a month during the free-offer periods.
6. The program was flexible, permitting action on field suggestions, and the free offers could be shifted according to demand, or moved seasonally, for example.
7. From a funding viewpoint, the study showed a way to pick up acceptances and use funds that might otherwise have been lost at the end of a budgetary year.

8. One area left unexplored was the possible negative diffusion effect on townships adjoining the *free* areas during the three month period. Workers complained, but little could be done to solve the problem, so little evaluation took place.

9. The project evolved from a two-township to a thirty-township approach, on a rotating basis to various areas, to a variety of free approaches (postpartum, etc.) — with the evaluation and program staff combining to get the fullest utilization potential from the results and to disseminate these to field workers to encourage their participation and enthusiasm.

SUGGESTIONS FOR DISCUSSION

1. Imagine that it is 1966 and that you are Mrs. Lin, the family planning field worker in Salu township, a rural fishing area in central Taiwan. You have been told that your town has been selected to have a three-month *free* IUD insertion offer starting in a month. As resources you have a desk and chair at the township health station (which provides some primary health care and has several nursing staff), a bicycle, expense money of about US$8 per month, some educational materials (posters and flyers), one private physician doing IUD insertions, an effective township birth registration office, and your imagination. Your normal working pattern is to visit women who have three children and get them interested in trying a contraceptive. Your visits are casual and you do about six to eight a day. There are about 5,000 women of childbearing ages in Salu, of whom about 20 per cent are currently using contraceptives. You work in Taichung County where there are twenty-four other workers in rural or suburban towns similar to yours. You will be meeting with the County Nurse and PPH Supervisors and these twenty-four workers at the monthly supervision meeting in Fengshan, the County Seat.

   How do you feel about the *free offer*? What could you do during this month to prepare for the offer? What do you plan to do differently in the field once the *free offer* starts?

2. How would you design a project that might separate the effect on increased IUD acceptances of the increased number of home visits a worker made during the *free offer* period from the effect of the public's reacting to the free offer itself? (See *Commentary* #1) Is it possible to design such a study? Why or why not? If you could separate the effect, what would be the educational program implications which could be applied in the field?

3. One foreign advisor speculated that the reason the field workers performed so actively during *free offer* periods was that they, for once, had bucked the bureaucracy and taken a measure of program control at the field level. Because the suggestion for the *free offer* was theirs (and their public's), it was given their best effort. How do you react to this idea? Are there applications for this to other health education programs you may be working on?

#6 — TODAY KAOHSIUNG, TOMORROW TAIWAN*

Summary • The Need for Action • The Campaign •
Results • Commentary • Suggestions for Discussion

SUMMARY

The Kaohsiung Study is frequently cited as an example of a pilot program which had a major effect on broadening the health education outputs of a large-scale family planning program. It also demonstrated to skeptics that it was possible to add another contraceptive method to program services without it adversely affecting the major method being provided. In a program where a huge majority of administrators and program advisors zealously and enthusiastically were devoted to the merits of the intrauterine contraceptive device, this change did not come about easily. To some extent, this study also relieved the anxiety of higher-level governmental officials who feared that public discussion of contraception through the mass media might cause public reaction, or worse, bring down the wrath of conservative legislators who had continued to oppose the Government's unofficial population policy and held back early governmental and quasi-governmental efforts at family planning. A euphemistically named "Pre-pregnancy Health" program providing face-to-face education at home or small group meetings was acceptable — so long as the workers were not officially government employees, so long as it was mostly private physicians who did IUD insertions, so long as the Taiwan Provincial Health Department only did education and the services were paid for by the quasi-voluntary organization (Maternal and Child Health Association) set up for this purpose. But a higher profile was considered undiplomatic without an official policy.

The Kaohsiung Study, which is discussed here, demonstrates the value of having clear-cut objectives, continuing feedback of results, and the cooperation of program administrators and applied research and evaluation staff in a single agency. It was on these resources that this communication study was built and which enabled it to serve as a model for rapid and successful expansion of the use of mass media in the Island-wide action-oriented family planning program.

THE NEED FOR ACTION

The record of experimentation in family planning is replete with examples of approaches that were first tried out in the experimental

---

*Expanded from research done with Laura Lu and T. H. Sun, both formerly with the Taiwan Committee on Family Planning, and funded by the Population Council and the East-West Communication Institute.

context and later adopted as policy . . . . The Kaohsiung mass study in Taiwan was the model for the island-wide mass communications campaign which began in 1972 [47].

1959-1964

The story of how this large-scale experiment was decided upon and implemented is a long one. To begin at a reasonable beginning, we need to go back no later than 1959 when "pre-pregnancy health" (PPH) services at local health stations in Taiwan were offering conventional contraceptives. We would move then to the classic Taichung Study (discussed in case form in this book) and then on to the IUD-centered family planning program begun on an island-wide basis in mid-1964. From the beginning, primarily because of the lack of an official government policy supporting family planning, the main emphasis of the information and education program had been face-to-face communication, carried out by home-visiting family planning workers. Mass media was limited by policy (until May 1968), a small budget, and almost no staff. Virtually, the only use of mass media prior to early 1966 was the limited distribution of news releases. The program was almost entirely home-visit oriented.

Late 1965

In fact, in December 1965, a survey of key local family planning program leaders and executors showed that the use of mass media had low priority among them, partly due to the lack of official policy but partly due to limited experience with the media.

Mid-1966

Restrictions on the use of mass media relaxed slightly in 1966 as it became evident to program administrators that many key government personnel supported family planning. By mid-1966, the key program planners were willing to try out an experimental approach on a small budget to see if mass media could increase acceptance rates. A major city to the south, Kaohsiung, was chosen as the pilot area. It was Taiwan's second largest city, with a population of more than 600,000, and was a rapidly growing industrial area. It was chosen for these reasons and because its contraceptive acceptance rate was one of the lowest of the island's twenty-two county and city areas.

THE CAMPAIGN

The objectives of the Kaohsiung study were to prepare for and evaluate a campaign to increase contraceptive practice in Kaohsiung by more active use of mass media, extensive use of this industrial area's organizational network, and increased staff effort. They also included introducing the pill to find out if it would adversely affect loop acceptances. Taiwan's program was almost exclusively IUD-centered and pill acceptances were limited to those who had discontinued the IUD or had contraindications to usage.

The study was planned by the Taiwan Committee on Family Planning with the Population Council, an international educational foundation which provided funds and advisory assistance for the family planning program. The Kaohsiung Health Bureau staff were involved early in the planning and later were responsible for program implementation. The Chief of the Education Division of the Committee and the resident education advisor of the Population Council designed the study. In terms of quasi-experimental design, it was basically a pretest although a matching area, Tainan County in the south, was monitored as a control (i.e., no mass media or widespread expansion of contraceptives were used). The dependent variable was primarily acceptance of contraceptives (IUD insertions and the oral contraceptives) since fertility could not be measured over a period of a year or two. Knowledge and attitude, of course, were measured and used as criteria of change. Knowledge and attitude, however, are often open to questions of validity in large-scale knowledge, attitude and practice (KAP) surveys.

Furthermore, experience had shown that hard-hearted program administrators were more likely to be impressed with increases in practice than knowledge or attitude. This thinking pattern caused difficulties for program researchers who thought more in the theoretical framework of mass media as being more useful in increasing awareness and knowledge than either attitudes or practice.

Late 1966

A random stratified sample survey of 1,500 wives was conducted in Kaohsiung in November 1966 to establish guidelines for carrying out the program. Questions about radio listening habits, movie attendance, newspaper and magazine reading, TV viewing, and attendance at public meetings revealed that the most promising forms of mass media were radio and movies. Questions about family planning knowledge, attitudes, and practice indicated that important groups to reach were the uneducated and those not wanting more children but not practicing contraception. These data were used in campaign design. The survey also served as a benchmark to measure the effect of the planned media campaign.

Early 1967

The campaign began in January 1967, using mass media to spread information about family planning. It lasted through most of 1967. The pill was offered to all wives in Kaohsiung, although its use in the rest of Taiwan was restricted to women who had discontinued the IUD.

May 1968

A follow-up survey in May 1968 of the wives interviewed in November 1966 was conducted to measure program impact. It determined:

1. the amount and types of exposure to family planning mass media and other public information;
2. changes in knowledge, attitudes, and practice of family planning, particularly with respect to the two program methods (the loop and the pill); and
3. the role the campaign played in promoting change.

Longer-term observation was used to determine if providing the pill to all wives who wanted it lowered the acceptances of the loop.

Generally speaking, the initial survey and field feedback provided a good idea of the educational content needed in the public information campaign. The over-all tendency was to stress the informational approach, rather than the motivational. For example, part of the campaign in Kaohsiung City was to gauge the response to the oral pill if all women who wished it were offered it at the low cost of ten NT dollars (US25¢) per cycle. Although some public information material had been prepared, reactions of the Taiwan women to the pill beyond that assessed in a few limited clinical or mailing studies was not known to any large extent. Responses to survey questions of those wives who had heard of the loop (about 62%) and of the oral pill (about 55%) were rather interesting in terms of planning a public information campaign. About 53 per cent of those who had heard of the loop knew one or more disadvantages of its use. This made it difficult for some program administrators to support the viewpoint sometimes expressed that it was better not to mention the possibility of minor side effects.

The pill also provided some more interesting considerations. Pamphlets received from the Western pill supplier stressed not worrying about weight gain with the oral pill. In calorie conscious western countries a few pounds more are considered a problem for women susceptible to gaining excess weight. This aesthetic consideration seemed to have little or no relevance to Taiwan's slenderer women. About 26 per cent of those interviewed who had heard of the pill knew some of its advantages — one being weight gain. A visit to a number of Taiwan's local health stations supported this finding. Many Taiwan women considered weight gain an advantage — a kind of "desirable side effect."

Ability to prevent pregnancy, difficulty in use, cost and the lack of or presence of certain kinds of side effects were both major advantages and disadvantages cited by respondents. These generally were integrated into the content of the public information material being prepared.

Prior to the pre-action survey in 1966, the family planning action program consisted of nineteen full-time field workers stationed at the ten district public health stations and offering only the loop. Following the survey, radio, movies, mailings, and selected industrial and other public organizations were harnessed to promote not only the loop but also the pill which was introduced on January 20, 1967. The price of each cycle of pills was set at NT$10 per cycle (US25¢), and all wives who wished it could have it (provided they had not been using it before).

The more intensive program input included among others the following actions which were not normally carried out at the time: fifty local physicians, nineteen local full-time PPH field workers, eight village health education nurses, and a large number of local health station and bureau staff received special orientation and training (and new PPH workers were recruited), particularly about the newly-introduced pill; supply depots for pills were set up at the ten district health stations and also at ten other clinics (four run by industrial organizations, four were military hospitals, two provincial and city hospitals); educational materials were provided to the ten health stations and ten clinics; PPH and VHEN workers held meetings for employees of large factories; and conducted evening outdoor film showings (for about six months); 1,558 letters offering free loop insertions for a limited time only were sent (from Taichung) to local Education Department employees (mainly teachers); 25,000 letters containing contraceptive information were sent to married couples working in local industry. About 5,000 plastic packets including both maternal and child health care and family planning information were distributed through the Provincial and City Government Hospital OBGYN wards. Furthermore, radio spot announcements were placed on two local radio stations in addition to those already on one Island-wide network for a period of about nine months, and a set of three colorful slides advertising the loop and pill were shown daily at three shows in twenty-eight movie theaters in the city for a three-month period.

RESULTS

Knowledge about family planning methods, particularly the IUD and pill, increased greatly. Citing of mass media as a source of information also increased greatly. There was considerable diffusion of information to others from those who received it directly. Current practice of contraception rose among the sample survey of wives from 33 per cent (pre-campaign) to 42 per cent afterward. Among the overall population, the introduction of the pill seems not to have detracted much from IUD acceptances, which rose by 16 per cent after the pill program began (1967) (see Table 5).

The program's conclusions were that the campaign was successful in increasing knowledge and acceptance of family planning methods and that the availability of the pill did not decrease acceptance levels for the IUD. Subsequent decisions by the island-wide family planning program directors to

Table 5. Average Monthly Loop Acceptors: 1965-1969

	1965	1966	Per Cent Increase 1965-1966	1967	Per Cent Increase 1966-1967	1968	Per Cent Increase 1967-1968	1969	Per Cent Increase 1968-1969
Taiwan Area	8,261	9,270	+12.2	10,045	+ 8.4	10,306	+2.6	10,863	+ 5.4
Kaohsiung City	354	374	+ 5.7	434	+16.0	468	+7.8	570	+21.8
Tainan County	536	729	+36.0	742	+ 1.8	729	-1.8	715	- 1.9

SOURCE: Cernada, G. and L. Lu, The Kaohsiung Study, Studies in Family Planning, 3:8, p. 203, August 1972.

use mass media and to introduce the pill throughout the island can in part be attributed to the success of their use in the Kaohsiung Study.

The final results of the intensive Kaohsiung project were dramatic enough to convince program administrators to begin use of mass media on a wider scale. As importantly, however, intermediate results were fed back to administrators as they became available, since loop and pill acceptor figures were produced monthly.

COMMENTARY

1. The overall Taiwan program for the first time acquired information on who listened to the radio, read newspapers or magazines, attended movies, and owned a TV, and on what programs were popular. These findings helped plan wiser use of public information expenditures in urban areas. They also served as leverage to gain more funding for public information.

   To help simplify the results for program administrators, charts were prepared and slides shown of the mass media audience profile. Reports and articles were mimeographed in early 1967 and circulated to help program leaders think about the potential for using mass media on a wider scale. These early results were fed back into the program as soon as they became available and geared into the interests of administrators — e.g., the Health Commissioner had expressed considerable interest in radio as a medium and the radio audience was emphasized particularly. Key administrators who had been concerned with the need to reach the poor and illiterate were provided breakdowns of this media audience (see Figure 10).

2. Staff increased their experience in producing public information materials, identifying audiences, budgeting for and dealing with mass media agencies, and organizing a concentrated effort, particularly with existing organizations

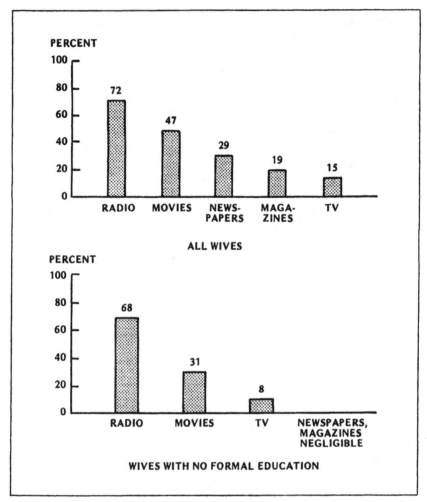

SOURCE: Cernada, G. and L. Lu, The Kaohsiung Study, *Studies in Family Planning*, 3:8, p. 199, August 1972.

Figure 10. Percentages of wives aged 20-44 reached by communication channels: all wives and wives with no formal education.

other than public health (factories, unions, industrial clinics). The need for an information/education section at program headquarters in Taichung became evident, and staff were drawn from the project to establish one.

3. The Study showed that public information channels, particularly mass media, can get family planning messages to wives at a comparatively low cost. This finding helped get the island-wide mass media campaign started later. Much skepticism existed about the affordability of mass media or whether they

could help bring couples to accept family planning. This skepticism was based on a strong orientation toward face-to-face approaches, which had been shown to produce results at low cost, from unfamiliarity with the media, the lack of public policy, and from a fear of diversion of funds from ongoing projects to mass media. Whenever possible, the findings were presented as showing that mass media would be a useful *supplement* to the existing field worker approach. Their relatively low cost was highlighted, as was the possibility of using existing government channels (i.e., radio stations, etc.) to carry out the task at no cost. As larger local budgets became available from 1968 on, the mass media became logical candidates for funding as regular program items.

Demonstrating the effect of the media was no easy task. To show its effect on the audience, evaluators spent a good deal of time treating matched cases, discussing ramifications of the pre- and post-surveys (e.g., possible effect of time as a confounding variable), the extent of diffusion beyond the recipients of the media messages, etc. (see Figure 11 and Tables 6, 7, and 8).

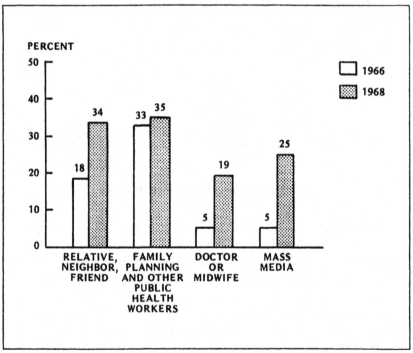

SOURCE: Cernada, G. and L. Lu, The Kaohsiung Study, *Studies in Family Planning*, 3:8, p. 202, August 1972.

Figure 11. All wives by percentages knowing of loop
by source of information: 1966 and 1968.

Table 6. Percentages of Wives Reached by
Family Planning Mass Media Approaches

Medium	Percentages Receiving Information by May 1968 Post-Survey	Percentages Receiving Information since November 1966 Pre-Survey
Radio	34.8	28.7
Mailings	17.4	15.1
Newspapers	17.3	11.2
Magazines	10.4	6.2
Movies	7.7	6.4
TV	2.4	2.0

SOURCE: Cernada, G. and L. Lu, The Kaohsiung Study, *Studies in Family Planning*, 3:8, p. 200, August 1972.

Table 7. Audience Reached by Mass Media: 1966 and 1968

Type of Information and Information Source	Preliminary Survey November 1966	As Per Cent of All Wives	Follow-up Survey May 1968	As Per Cent of All Wives
Per cent of those knowing of any method citing mass media as source	27	(24)	45	(42)
Per cent of those knowing of loop citing mass media as source	9	(5)	37	(24)
Per cent of those knowing of pill citing mass media as source	23	(13)	25[a]	(14)
Per cent of all wives knowing of family planning through radio	—	25.2	—	34.8
Per cent of all wives who received family planning mailings	—	1.5[b]	—	17.4

SOURCE: Cernada, G. and L. Lu, The Kaohsiung Study, *Studies in Family Planning*, 3:8, p. 201, August 1972.

[a] Although mass media sources did not rise much from 1966 for the pill, 7 per cent of all wives had heard about it from the PPH or public health staff compared to less than 1 per cent in 1966 — an indication of another aspect of the program effort.

[b] Mailings did not begin until April 1966. No commercial sources carried out mailings.

Table 8. Diffusion of Information by Percentage Among All Wives

Medium	Learning of Family Planning News in Media from Others	Receiving Family Planning News Directly from Media	Learning from Both Sources
Radio	26.2	34.8	21.2
Newspapers	25.0	17.3	12.4
Magazines	11.6	10.4	7.3
Mailings	8.9	17.4	5.3
Movies	6.5	7.7	4.0
TV	2.9	2.4	1.6

SOURCE: Cernada, G. and L. Lu, The Kaohsiung Study, *Studies in Family Planning*, 3:8, p. 201, August 1972.

Due to a series of problems, the finished detailed analysis was not completed until mid-1970, or nearly two years after the post-survey was completed. However, the need to demonstrate results conclusively (i.e., the effect of media on acceptance) had become academic because the program administrators had by then begun an education unit which was carrying out a modest mass media effort (based on the interim results and their actual participation in the Kaohsiung action program). By the end of 1967 it had become apparent that the low cost of about $2,000 for the added mass media input and increased field worker input had produced an increase in loop acceptances by 12 per cent in 1967 versus 9 per cent island-wide, plus a doubling of total acceptances (if the pill is included) over the previous year.

4. Effective programs demand effective planning. To plan, information affecting the planned program's implementation is needed. For mass media, audience surveys are a must. Because of this pre-campaign survey, administrators became more aware of the need to have the overall program evaluation staff routinely gather information on mass media and public information channels. Prior to the Kaohsiung Survey, island-wide sample KAP surveys had largely ignored gathering information on the composition of the mass media audience. This lack of action partially reflected the heavy emphasis on fertility rather than the knowledge or attitude components in the surveys. A series of questions based on and expanded from the Kaohsiung surveys was added to subsequent KAP studies and greater attention began to be paid to evaluation of the mass communication component of the program, particularly use of media. Analysis of media findings became routine with brief interim reports prepared for circulation to key concerned staff.

5. Providing oral contraceptives to all who wanted them (and who had no contraindications to use) in the study seems not to have affected loop referrals. The island-wide program had avoided giving the pill to all wives

who wanted it from the fear that it would lower loop acceptances. In late 1970, partly due to the Kaohsiung findings, the pill was made available to all who wanted it and were screened for contraindications to use.

To keep administrators posted, there were regular reports issued. Detailed records of acceptors were kept on a monthly basis at each health station in Kaohsiung City. Although it was clear by 1968 that the pill was not lowering loop acceptances (the rural study in Tainan also demonstrated this), it was not until two years after the 1968 post-survey that the program took action to remove restrictions and provide pills to all wives who wanted them. Two factors combined to postpone change. One was the existing program attitudes about the role of the pill as a supplementary method (due to lower use continuation than with the IUD); the other was the fear that the free supply of pills might come to an end, and funds would not be available to provide supplies to a larger number of women (some of whom would have been switching from commercial brands). The study results were clear, but it took time for these to counter previously existing attitudes.

6. The study results were instrumental in getting funding to broaden mass media use, first from the Population Council (which was involved heavily in the Kaohsiung experiment) and then from the government.

In summary, the Kaohsiung Study illustrated the value of:

1. Action-oriented, evaluative communication research carried out within one agency so that action can be taken based upon results. (Imagine how much less likely it would have been for results to have been applied on such a large scale had an outside agency carried out this project!)
2. Quick feedback of results into the program, particularly geared to administrators in their own frames of references (see the figures and tables).
3. Integration of mass media audience assessment into future surveys in order to continue collecting data which permit comparison. Without this integration into the national KAP surveys, the later national shift in audience attention from radio to TV might have been less noticeable or not observed so soon.
4. The cooperative effort of program and evaluation staff: program action staff implementing the project based upon their years of field experience and the evaluation staff[1] assisting in selecting a random sample for survey, and helping draft pre- and post-program questionnaires [48].

SUGGESTIONS FOR DISCUSSION

1. A difficulty of adapting educational materials from one culture to the other is illustrated well by the Kaohsiung pre-campaign survey. Much of the Western literature on oral contraceptives dealt with weight gain as a side

[1] Taiwan Population Studies Center.

effect which would be viewed negatively by women. In Taiwan, the survey showed that women viewed a slight weight gain as a "positive" side-effect. What other examples of difficulties in cross-cultural transference of ideas are you familiar with? From your own experience? From your readings in this book?

2. This case study emphasizes the merits of having the research and evaluation units, in effect, as part of the same organization as the program planning and implementation units. What do you think are the relative disadvantages of such an organizational arrangement? To what extent do you think the arrangement may limit the objectivity of the evaluating unit?

3. As you will note in the case study, the authors indicate that program administrators want action/practice results, not just changes in knowledge and attitude. To what extent does this thinking pattern influence how health education programs are conducted? How do you think that it may have influenced the Kaohsiung campaign? Its evaluation? To what extent should the effectiveness of health education programs be judged by behavioral changes? What are the dangers of "blaming the victim" if only informational campaigns are pursued to bring about change?

4. The Kaohsiung Study is referred to as a quasi-experiment. Do you understand the difference between an experimental design and a quasi-experimental one? Why are "true" experimental designs difficult to conduct in the world outside the laboratory?

5. Would it have been possible to design the Kaohsiung Study to totally separate the effects of the mass media from the other accelerated program inputs? Would it have been worthwhile if it were possible?

#7 — INCENTIVES: BEYOND FAMILY PLANNING*

Summary • The Need for Action • Results •
Commentary • Suggestions for Discussion

SUMMARY

This case study* describes two truly innovative research projects which had as their major educational objective, calling attention of the Government to the need and possibility of providing positive incentives for having fewer children than the norm — and deriving considerable cost benefit in terms of the social and economic values of births averted and satisfaction with smaller families. These projects also were part of a regional Asian, indeed international, plan to introduce the concept of moving beyond the bounds of conventional family planning programs which emphasized education about childbearing and provision of contraceptive services almost exclusively.

The two studies, the Huatan Educational Savings Plan and the Taichung Birth Spacing Incentive Plan began in March 1971 and March 1975 respectively. Both were based on previous research findings and program observation. The latter attempted to incorporate some of the early lessons learned in the former. The purpose of the Educational Savings Plan was to provide financial support for the future education of children of parents whose families did not go beyond three children. The Taichung Spacing Incentive Plan was to encourage younger women to prolong the interval between first and second births to at least three years by providing education and an incentive of free delivery services (or a cash equivalent) for the second child. Both succeeded in demonstrating the possibility of use of incentives and a great deal was learned about the kind of unanticipated problems which can arise from long-term and innovative projects of this sort.

This case also illustrates:

1. how previous research results were utilized in planning and guiding these programs;

2. how foreign aid, otherwise unobtainable, was made possible because the plan was innovative and had regional implications; and

*Written by George P. Cernada and T.H. Sun. Expanded from a more brief version by the authors concentrating only on the Educational Savings Plan appearing in *Papers of the East-West Communication Institute*, No. 10, July 1974. Part of the Huatan program description relies heavily upon articles by Finnigan and Sun [49], and Wang and Chen [50]. The projects described were carried out by the Taiwan Provincial Institute of Family Planning. The Educational Savings Plan was designed by T. H. Sun and O. D. Finnigan and the Taichung Spacing Incentive Plan by T. H. Sun and G. Cernada.

3. some of the problems about how to influence national leaders to take more widespread action based on these programs.

THE NEED FOR ACTION

1969

The crude birth rate had declined from a 1951 peak of fifty to about twenty-eight per thousand. Although the family planning program was providing extensive services to meet public demand, program administrators became concerned that the birth rate might not only stop declining but even rise. This concern was caused by survey findings and analysis of fertility data which showed that:

1. an unusually large number of young people were entering the reproductive years;
2. the fertility of young women continued to be high;
3. there had been little change in the number of children wanted by each couple;
4. a strong son preference continued to prevail, which influenced some couples to produce a larger number of children than they wanted; and
5. the fertility of women aged thirty and above who had already had enough children was very low. (See Figure 12.)

In summary, women who had had their ideal number of children were effective in controlling their fertility and further fertility decline depended largely on a change in ideal family size (number of children in particular and probably number of sons). These factors, which came under consideration in 1968 after the government support for family planning became official, led program administrators to think about how to educate couples to the advantages of having fewer children.

Administrators asked the program's research and evaluation unit to find out why families wanted so many children and to try to develop incentives as compensation. At this time it would have been difficult if not impossible to get local funding for such an innovative project due to a lack of funds and for political reasons. Taiwan also had "graduated" from American aid in 1965 and the door to direct funding from that source was closed. Since this important problem had regional implications, however, Taiwan was able to obtain a grant from the Population Council (using AID funds) in 1970 for several innovative projects which were developed to try to find answers to the problem.

Educational Savings Plan

Although the studies proposed relating to incentives were more exploratory in the funding proposal, the actualization was the Educational Savings Plan.

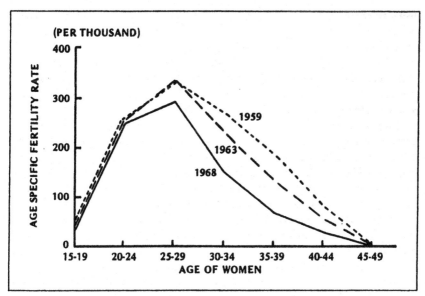

SOURCE: *Taiwan's Family Planning in Charts*, 3rd ed., Taiwan Provincial Institute of Family Planning, p. 56, 1969.

Figure 12. Change in age-specific fertility.
(The 1968 curve shows that younger women ages 25-29 are showing some drop in fertility and have been since 1965. The fertility decline between 1959 and 1963, though, was entirely due to women 30 and older. Since the number of women 20-24 will increase by 60 per cent by 1973, greater effort must be made to reach these younger women. Other agencies than public health also must contribute.)

This was later followed by the Taichung Spacing Incentives Plan, but not for four years. The Educational Savings Plan was based heavily on previous research. In Taiwan, it had been considered important to have many children in order to provide for old-age support. A 1969 survey of men found that 62 per cent expected to live with their children in old age and 57 per cent expected money from time to time regardless of the children's economic condition. These findings are consistent with traditional Chinese values: the extended family pattern with expectation for old-age support as the rationale for wanting and having large families, with more sons. On the average, couples wanted 2.3 sons and 1.6 daughters. The desire for sons also reflects other deep-rooted cultural values in a Confucian-oriented society where continuation of family name and ancestral worship are linked to male progeny. In societies where the death rate is high, the number of children wanted includes enough to make up for expected deaths. In Taiwan, however, medical care, public health services and rising living standards had reduced the death rate to less than five per thousand. There also was an effective, island-wide contraceptive delivery system. Most of the couples in Taiwan seemed to be confident (though fears persisted that they would be the exception) that their children would live, and they have achieved their expected fertility with relative ease. As of 1970, the "average" woman wanted 3.9 children; total fertility averaged 4.0. Forty-four per cent of married women aged twenty to forty-four were practicing contraception in 1970.

These findings lead to the question of how Taiwanese expect their children to succeed financially. Surveys indicated that parents perceive the path to financial success to be through education. Traditionally, Chinese families have strongly emphasized higher education and commercial or professional employment. Although only 16 per cent of men have attended high school or college, 67 per cent expect one or more of their children to finish college. And although only 29 per cent have any idea of the cost of a college education, 76 per cent say that this will be a "heavy financial burden." When asked whether saving money is important, 78 per cent say that it is, and, among these, 40 per cent spontaneously cite the cost of education as the most important reason for saving. These conditions became the base for developing the educational incentive savings program in 1971. The program capitalized on the strong desire to save by establishing for the couple who limits family size a bank account earmarked for education for children. The program deposited money for the couple who succeeded in limiting children to two or three. The account, which was to help cover high school and college tuition and fees, was expected to provide schooling from junior high through senior high.

1971

Huatan, a rural township in Changhua County, located in the middle part of the west coast of the island, was selected for the pilot project. This township had a population of about 35,000, with 1,477 married women less than thirty years old with three or fewer children listed in the town registration office. These women were eligible for the program. In actuality, only 1,103 of them were still living in Huatan when a baseline survey took place. Of these, 1,051 were interviewed in mid-1971, but ninety either did not complete the interview or were pregnant for the fourth time. Thus, the final population to be followed in this study was 961. Results confirmed prior island-wide findings reported earlier. The mean desired number of children was 3.5, with a decided preference for sons. Although only 26 per cent of husbands and 9 per cent of wives had attended junior high school or above, almost 75 per cent expected sons and over 50 per cent expected daughters to finish college. Sixty-five per cent expected to live with their children for the rest of their lives, and 64 per cent felt that their children should give them money regardless of the child's economic condition. Although 95 per cent felt that it was necessary to save money and over half of

Table 9. Summary of Preliminary Survey Findings, Hua-tan Township,
Per Cent Among Married Women Under Age Thirty with
Three or Fewer Children (N = 961)

A. COMPLETED EDUCATION

| | Actual | | Expected for Children | |
	Wife	Husband	Son(s)	Daughter(s)
Primary or Below	91	74	6	16
Junior or Senior High	8	23	23	30
College or Other	1	3	71	54
	100	100	100	100

B. SAVINGS

Beliefs About		Practice in Recent Years	
Very Necessary to Save	79	Save Regularly	9
Necessary to Save	16	Save Occasionally	27
Not Necessary to Save	5	Never Save	64
	100		100

C. EXPECTATIONS OF CHILDREN

Expect to Live with Them		Expect Money from Them	
For Rest of Life	65	In All Cases	64
When Old	4	If Live Together	2
Depends on Situation	23	Depends on Situation	21
No	8	No	13
	100		100

SOURCE: O. D. Finnigan and T. H. Sun, Planning, Starting, and Operating an Educational Incentive Project, *Studies in Family Planning*, 3:1, p. 3, 1972.

these felt that the primary purpose of saving was for education, only 9 per cent had saved regularly in recent years and 64 per cent had never saved anything (see Table 9). These findings helped support the rationale of the plan.

The actual plan underwent a number of revisions, partially based on funding limitations and difficulties in estimating the long-term rate of inflation and its effect on educational costs. A description of the plan follows.

> In its final form the pilot project offers to couples with zero, one, or two children an annual deposit in a savings account for each year that they do not exceed two living children. These deposits are recorded on an account card kept by each enrolled woman. If a

couple has a third child, the value of the savings account is immediately reduced by 50 per cent. If they have a fourth child, it is cancelled and all funds are returned to the bank.

The account is held at the maximum permissible long-term interest rate (now 9.5 per cent), and all accumulated interest is added to the account. The enrollment deposit is large enough to be attractive to most couples, and annual deposits increase as the program progresses. The account can be closed by a one-time withdrawal from ten to fourteen full years after enrollment. At this time a book of cashier's checks will be issued payable for educational expenses in public high schools and colleges, and equal to the total amount of deposits plus interest. After ten full years the account will be worth US$267.50. If the couple waits for four additional years, the account increases in value by $117.10 to $384.60 [51].

The deposit schedule and estimated account value at withdrawal are described in Table 10.

Table 10. Educational Savings Plan Deposit and Withdrawal Schedules at 9.5 Per Cent Interest Compounded Annually (U.S. Dollars)

A. REGULAR PLAN			B. SPECIAL PLAN	
	Annual Deposits			Annual Deposits
Year	0-2 Children	3 Children	Year	3 Children
0	$ 25.00	$ 12.50	0	$ 35.00
1	5.00	2.50	1	7.50
2	5.00	2.50	2	7.50
3	10.00	5.00	3	10.00
4	10.00	5.00	4	10.00
5	15.00	7.50	5	12.50
6	15.00	7.50	Total	$ 82.50
7	20.00	10.00		
8	20.00	10.00		
9	25.00	12.50		
10	25.00	12.50		
Total	$175.00	$ 87.50		
	Value of Account at Withdrawal			Value of Account at Withdrawal
Year	0-2 Children	3 Children	Year	3 Children
10	$267.50	$133.75	6	$133.75
11	292.96	146.48	7	146.48
12	320.80	160.40	8	160.40
13	351.24	175.62	9	175.62
14	384.60	192.30	10	192.30

SOURCE: O. D. Finnigan and T. H. Sun, Planning, Starting, and Operating an Educational Incentive Project, Studies in Family Planning, 3:1, p. 2, 1972.

A special plan was offered to couples who already had three children. Deposits are increased and the savings account matures from six to ten years after deposits begin, payable at the reduced rate used for all other three-child families. This plan aims at attracting quickly couples before they have a fourth child.

Spacing Incentive Plan

Many of the staff of the Taiwan Provincial Institute of Family Planning long had been criticized by colleagues and counterparts in Taipei because Taichung City, where the Institute was headquartered, was not among the highest geographic areas in terms of contraceptive practice. When an experiment was suggested to test out whether incentives could be provided to reward couples who spaced between births for a minimum of three years, it was natural to consider Taichung as the setting. Furthermore, the program had historical precedent for selecting the difficult geographic areas to prove its point (e.g., Kaohsiung City for the mass media demonstration project). Taichung also had a large population base so that results would appear more impressive in a population of as large as half a million. And last, but not least, the program would be directly at hand in a city where most of the staff worked, played, and lived.

This project began not only as a means of testing incentives but also as a way of reaching younger women who, as indicated earlier, had high fertility rates and were increasing greatly in numbers. Studies had shown that child spacing was not being encouraged by the family planning program which emphasized limitation. Furthermore, the average interval between marriage and first child had shortened from sixteen months in 1970 (indeed, by 1976, it was twelve months). The interval between first and second child which had been thirty months in 1970 also was growing smaller (indeed, by 1976, it had gone down to only twenty-four months). In Taichung City in 1971 the mean interval between first and second child was 26.4 months (see Table 11). It was clear also that since so many pregnancies began before the marriages were registered, reaching newlyweds to postpone a first birth would be a difficult task (as results of a Newlywed Project earlier had indicated). It was decided, therefore, to try to reach women under thirty years old with one child. The objectives of the project, as stated in the original funding proposal (see Appendix D) were as follows:

1. To carry out an action plan in Taichung City (capital city of the Province of Taiwan) to enroll all couples, after the birth of their first child, in an educational and incentive-oriented program to promote expanding the mean open birth interval from the *present mean of 23.7 months to 36, 42, or 48 months and beyond.*
2. To reward all those who enroll by providing free contraceptives and additional educational services. For those who reach three years without a birth, free delivery service for their second child (as well as hospital ca:·

Table 11. Percentage Distribution of Wives by Open Length of
Second Live Birth Intervals: Taichung City (1970)[a]

Age	No./Wives	No Birth	0-6	6-12	12-18	18-24	24-30	30+
				Per Cent Wives in Each Interval				
22-29	64	37.5	0	4.7	10.9	20.3	15.6	10.9
30-42	107	0.9	0	0	19.6	32.7	20.6	26.2
22-42	171	14.6	0	1.8	16.4	28.1	18.7	20.5

Mean length of open interval: 23.7 months (ages 22-29)
27.4 months (ages 30-42)
26.4 months (ages 22-42)

SOURCE: Taiwan Provincial Institute of Family Planning.

[a] This computation is based upon the 171 Taichung City wives who had a first live birth in the island-wide sample KAP survey (1970).

and other services for those who continue longer without a second child) will be provided.

3. For the Taiwan Provincial Health Department to demonstrate to the Taiwan Provincial Government that this service is (a) worth providing on a larger scale due to its maternal health and demographic values, and (b) easily duplicable by having public Provincial and County Hospitals (now under the authority of the Provincial Health Department and Taiwan Provincial Government) provide this free delivery and maternity care.

4. To expand the project at the end of two years to include similar incentives (a) for postponing marriage, (b) for postponing a first child for a minimum of two years, (c) for continuing periods of non-fertility after the second child.

It was hoped that this project could bring the mean interval between the first and second child from 23.7 to about 42 months or almost double the time length for 1971. A copy of the project proposal is included as Appendix D for those wishing to refer to it.

To get the funding, which was difficult to secure locally, the project proposal emphasized its international demonstration value. (It may be worth noting that a long-time major donor, The Population Council, was phasing out its funding so that this resource was unavailable.) Such an incentive would seem to be more likely to be acceptable to African or Latin American countries where encouragement of child spacing would be politically more acceptable than incentives for not bearing a third or fourth child. Funding for the study was provided by the International Committee for Applied Research on Population (ICARP) and the project got underway in March 1975. All married women below thirty years of age as of January 1, 1974, registered as residents in Taichung City and having had a first child born between April 1, 1974 and March 31, 1975, were eligible to enroll.

RESULTS

Educational Savings Plan

September 1971 — Sixty-seven per cent of the 1,089 eligible couples joined the program. Among those 728 who joined, 541 had two or fewer children (regular plan) and 187 had three children (three-child plan). As expected, enrollment was highest among women who (in a pre-survey) indicated that they wanted no more children (79%), already were using contraception (82%), or had as many sons as they wanted (75%). Other social and economic variables such as income, education, occupation, or aspirations for children seemed not to be significant predictors of enrollment, probably due to the active recruiting by village administrators of eligible women for enrollment.

Later 1971 — A series of mini-surveys was conducted after the first enrollment to find out:

1. if the enrollment brought about increased contraceptive practice or intention of further contraceptive practice (mini-survey no. 1);
2. why some women failed to enroll in the program (mini-survey no. 2); and
3. to interview women who became pregnant after enrollment (no. 3).

Survey findings were used in introducing supplemental actions to keep the enrollees in the program. For example:

1. a name list of women who were not using contraception was given to the local family planning worker for follow-up;
2. free sterilization was offered to those who wished to have it; and
3. another chance to enroll in the program was given in 1972 to women who had failed to enroll in 1971 (more than half of them indicated that they might join the program in the future if given another chance).

September 1972 — Re-enrollment took place in September 1972, one year after the first enrollment. The result was registration of 96 per cent or 99 per cent when out-migrations and divorced couples were discounted. Forty-eight cases dropped out. Of the 361 eligible couples who did not enroll in 1971, fifty-seven enrolled in 1972. Partly due to limited funds, recruitment of new enrollees was not pressed, and no bonuses or prizes were given for new enrollment. An interview of the eight 1971 enrollees who were still eligible but had not re-enrolled in 1972 brought three of them to re-enroll in the three-child plan.

September 1973 — The re-enrollment a year later was 94 per cent: 690 of the eligible couples. Forty couples had a fourth child and dropped out, and seven either moved out or were unwilling to continue.

September 1980 — Nine years later, 174 of the original 728 couples who enrolled in the project remained. Some, however, had graduated on December 28, 1977 in a unique ceremony: 210 couples who had stayed in the project fo six years without having an additional child, or either husband or wife had had a sterilization, received a substantial cash payment. These couples had chosen to receive cash instead of waiting until 1981 when the project was due to end.

This project received a great deal of international publicity. Its major flaw was not being able to calculate how inflation would make the educational subsidy limited in value. A great deal, however, was learned. Another township nearby is being studied as a control. The birth records for eligible women both in the study and control townships are being reviewed. Analysis of the individual fertility data by cohort and parity is in progress. It does seem, though, that the project was feasible and could be replicated elsewhere if incentives can be made large enough to cover future educational prices. How to successfully maintain staff and township interest and enthusiasm over a decade, however, remains unanswered.

Spacing Incentive Plan

1975 — Prior to the enrollment, the incentive project was announced in the newspapers, on the radio, and by posters. Health station staff visited homes to explain the project. Meetings were held with local leaders. Mailings were sent. Free delivery at a public hospital was offered to women who postponed their second child for three years. If they preferred they could have a cash bonus of NT$700-NT$900 (US$19.50-US$25): NT$700 for spacing for three years, NT$800 for three and one-half years, and NT$900 for four years. As of March 31, 1975, 67 per cent of the 3,566 eligible women had enrolled. When those who were not at the addresses provided at the City District Registration offices were excluded, the enrollment rate was 79 per cent or quite close to the original target.

On the other hand, in their enthusiasm to get as large an enrollment as possible some workers appear to have signed up individuals who had not much interest in spacing births. Since incentives were provided to workers to enroll people and also to people to enroll, there was a good deal of stimulus to get people in. The matter of enrolling even those not truly interested was debated by headquarters and field staff from not only an education view ("Once involved, there will be some commitment and we can better teach them with educational stimuli. Not only that, those ones not wanting to space are the ones we really need to educate.") but from an evaluative view ("If too many not interested are signed up, then they will drop out easily and we will not know if the program works").

1976 — Those signing up were home visited and mailed health educational materials every three months (on baby and child care, contraceptive methods, immunizations, post-partum care, breast feeding, and child-spacing). They also were provided with small discounts at certain stores by showing their enrollment cards. At the end of one year, the women were visited by health workers. Of those who had enrolled, 71 per cent remained with the program (excluding those who moved out or who could not be located after three visits). Among those still enrolled, 76 per cent were using some form of contraception (and seven of ten of these using reliable methods such as the intrauterine contraceptive device, the oral contraceptive or condoms). Those disqualified included those who had withdrawn voluntarily, become pregnant, or had a child. At the end of a year, the situation although not overly optimistic was at least promising.

1977-1978 — By the end of the second year, 550 persons or 39 per cent of those who had re-enrolled the year before were still in the program excluding those who moved out or who could not be located after three visits). The continuation rate after two years was lower than what the program anticipated. The analysis of what this meant was further complicated by the large per cent of previous enrollees who were reported as having moved (23%). The per cent of pregnancies among those followed up also was higher than expected (35%).

By the end of the third year, 45 per cent of those who had re-enrolled the year before were still in the program (excluding those who moved or who could not be located).

30 December 1978 — The Taichung City Health Bureau held a tea party for the 265 "graduates" of the program who had successfully carried out their child spacing for three years or more. Their experiences were discussed and many useful suggestions were made about increasing the educational component of the program. Each graduate was awarded the cash incentive and a certificate praising her achievement.

March 1979 — There were 291 graduates of the program when it terminated in March 1979. It was clear that at least some persons would space their births under the auspices of the project. The number of graduates, however, was less than originally anticipated. Moreover, it was difficult to know what to make of the results since so many persons who enrolled were lost to follow-up. If, however, we consider the potential pool of all eligibles in Taichung City when the program began to have been 2,998, those graduating at the end of three years were only about 10 per cent. Of those who enrolled initially (2,373), they represent about 13 per cent or one of eight persons who enrolled and completed their three years of spacing. How unrealistic the original pre-implementation expectations of success were may be seen from the project proposal's goal of 60 per cent graduates. In terms of birth intervals, the average interval for 240 women who had succeeded in the program was fifty months. The average interval of women who did enroll was about 25 months. For comparison, in 1970 (see Table 11), 13 per cent of Taichung's women twenty-two to twenty-nine had had open second live birth intervals of thirty or more months. A comparison with Tainan City (in Southern Taiwan) which was used as a control however, showed little difference between the two areas. The degree to which Tainan served as an adequate control remains unsettled. Evaluation, of the project, therefore, continues.

COMMENTARY

Both of these projects are, in effect, completed. Their success or failure remains open to interpretation. In retrospect, there are a number of questions which remain to be answered about incentives and the need for a continuing educational effort to support such longer-term program maintenance. Perhaps the clearest is that the budgets provided for both Huatan and Taichung were minimal even at the time of program inception. As years went by, inflation greatly decreased the buying power of the incentives. Possibly some kind of inflation or cost of living index would have helped. The free delivery at a government hospital might have had more meaning outside of a large urban area which was progressing rapidly economically at the time. Or, if private physicians, who had been involved successfully in the Taichung Study and the latter Island-wide family planning program, could have been subsidized to provide free delivery, their popularity might have helped. Its successful application to a less developed country also is more likely.

In terms of dissemination of results internationally, maximum publicity was provided to the Educational Savings Plan. Relatively less went to the Spacing Incentive Plan which although a larger-scale project, began much later when Taiwan was only one among many ongoing and active family planning programs and was somewhat more isolated diplomatically. Furthermore, little was written about it and nothing published. In terms of national dissemination of information about the projects, both received a fair amount of publicity but neither assumed too high a profile. One obstacle to expansion was that implementing program staff felt that it was unlikely that either project would show dramatic results and that the likelihood of expansion on a larger scale was minimal. The logistics of managing the projects, the intensive resources necessary for education, and the prohibitive costs made expansion unlikely. Possibly the strongest advocates of these two projects were the Family Planning Institute's director and two foreign resident advisors and the enthusiasm shared by others wore off as the advisors who had helped design the projects left Taiwan. On the other hand, both of these projects were designed on a transfer system so that in theory at least no funds for incentives on a national scale would have left the government system.

Educational Savings Plan

In terms of this project's potential for further utilization there are both weak and strong points.

1. An economic analysis is needed to show the savings of the program in order to counter the contention that the plan would be too expensive to expand. The plan should stress the transfer payment nature of such a large-scale incentive program in which no funds actually leave the

government system (funds going directly from finance departments to a postal savings account of a couple and then to the education department).

2. This project built on research indicating the high value parents place on education of their children. More attention needs to be given to alternate incentive schemes — even the testing of alternate schemes on a competitive basis. This alternate testing was originally considered but bypassed to carry out the educational savings approach and in effect speed up the process toward establishing a "proven success" in non-fertility incentives. This faster start helped more other countries to become aware that a strong "beyond family planning" project was continuing in Asia. The "information diffusion" element was judged most important. Limited funding held back testing of more than one alternative until the Taichung Spacing Incentive in 1974.

3. This approach came about through a desire to be innovative enough in a series of projects so that they would have regional implications. A plan to test alternate forms of incentives was submitted to a donor agency in 1969 and approved. Had this potential monetary kind of encouragement for innovative research not been there (and had Taiwan not had a long history of use of acceptor and worker incentives) it would have been difficult to convince the policymakers to submit this early incentive testing proposal, which represented a dramatic advance by moving into the area of testing of alternate non-fertility incentives. With the funding available for a test of alternate non-fertility incentives, the atmosphere was conducive to beginning the Educational Savings Plan, which was carried out instead of the earlier plan.

4. In terms of the project's potential for expansion locally, there also were weak and strong points. Initially, in 1970, the project was set up through a voluntary agency without official government support and entirely with foreign funding. Later, in 1972, in an attempt to involve government officials, the Taiwan Provincial Commissioners of Health and of Social Affairs were asked to co-author the first year's report. This move helped strengthen the government "commitment." The problem, however, is that high level government officials change quickly: a problem for longer-term experimental projects.

Spacing Incentive Plan

1. Although results have been mixed, some variation or modification could be of considerable value to countries where primary health care and family planning programs are weak. Offering free delivery by a qualified individual (e.g., trained midwife) and contraceptives to space (rather than limit) births could be more politically acceptable and in line with broader social development planning in some African and perhaps South American countries.

2. In retrospect, both increased educational inputs and increased access to contraception would have helped. Furthermore, both cultural tradition and modernization were interacting to hamper program goals. For example, the Chinese Year of the Dragon, when a son is particularly desirable, fell into the three-year program period and all Taiwan's birth rate jumped dramatically. In addition, rapid economic development was attracting many women into the labor market again after marriage and having the preferred number of children early was a trend.

3. More emphasis ought to be placed on the original transfer system of payment which kept the funds involved within the governmental system. The transfer in this system is of a subsidy from units of one governmental agency (Health Department): from the Family Planning Institute to the Governmental hospitals providing delivery.

4. The educational approach to expanding birth intervals in this project needs to be carefully examined. Although expansion of the incentive may not be possible, the theme of a three-year interval between births is being integrated into the overall public health program. In 1977 an Island-wide spacing incentive began. Instead of free delivery, the 36,713 couples enrolling over three years were eligible for a semi-annual lottery with major electrical appliances as prizes. The effects now are being evaluated under an ICARP grant. Perhaps most importantly, the Taiwan program needs to reach men and women while they are in school to make them aware of the values of spacing and limiting children and of the equal value of sons and daughters. Then educational campaigns and incentive schemes will be able to build upon a more solid foundation.

SUGGESTIONS FOR DISCUSSION

1. What ethical issues are there in the use of incentives? For birth control? Why are these particularly important in less developed countries?

2. What do you view as strengths of the research utilization process involved in the Huatan Educational Savings Plan? In the Taichung Spacing Incentives Plan?

3. Why are these pilot programs described as "beyond family planning"? What other such programs have you heard of in other countries?

4. Why do you think Taiwan was so concerned with regional and international replication of studies and disseminating information abroad on innovative projects and their results?

5. Try to list the educational objectives of these two projects. How would you design an appropriate evaluation of the educational inputs into either or both?

6. How do you feel about whether either one of the projects was a "success" or not? By what criteria are you measuring success? Do you include the process as well as the outcome?

7. How might these projects have built up a stronger community base of support?

#8 — SCIENTIFIC AMERICAN GOES ASIAN*

Summary • Determining Research Needs • The Classic
Taichung Study • Use of the Results • Documentation and
Dissemination • Commentary • Suggestions for Discussion

SUMMARY

The setting is the capital of the Province of Taiwan in 1963-
1964. The case study deals with the classic Taichung Study. It shows:

1. how an action-oriented research program was organized, and how it
served as the base for expansion to the rest of Taiwan;
2. what kind of organizational setup and approaches expedited getting the
research results used; and
3. how the results were utilized to pass the word to other countries that
people were interested in controlling the number of children they would
have and would take action if the means were made available.

DETERMINING RESEARCH NEEDS

By 1963, Taiwan had made remarkable progress in eradicating
the diseases that killed. The reduction of the crude death rate from 18.2 to 5.5
in eighteen years speaks for itself. Its population growth rate, however, was 3
per cent and at that rate the population would double in size in about twenty
years. With a population of already nearly thirteen million, of whom less than
half were in the economically productive ages twenty to sixty-four, and a
population density of about 900 persons per square mile (about the third most
densely populated in the world), the potential problem was becoming recognized
by alert leaders. The Joint (Sino-American) Commission on Rural
Reconstruction (JCRR), being aware of the rapid population growth problems,
began to stimulate and assist government agencies, such as the Taiwan Provincial
Government, especially the Health Department, to initiate an informal family
planning program. It also assisted in establishing the Taiwan Population Studies
Center (TPSC) in the Provincial Health Department in 1961, with financial
assistance from the Population Council of New York and technical collaboration
of the Population Studies Center of the University of Michigan. One of the

* Written by George P. Cernada and T. H. Sun.

objectives of the TPSC was to survey the fertility behavior of Taiwanese women so that actions could be taken to reduce fertility. Previously, there had been no large-scale family planning activities except a small-scale "pre-pregnancy health" (PPH) program in Nantou County and the limited activities of the Family Planning Association of China, a voluntary agency. The contraceptive methods used were conventional. Several key Chinese health officials, especially the JCRR Rural Health Director and the Provincial Health Commissioner, felt that a larger effort was desirable. None of their staff, however, had experience or knew how to proceed with a large-scale family planning program. Therefore, a U.S.-based educational foundation, the Population Council, was consulted to help conduct a pilot project that would test the feasibility of a more intensive field program. Arrangements were made for the University of Michigan Population Studies Center to provide consultation for the TPSC to conduct the necessary research.

A sample survey covering the city of Taichung was planned to measure women's knowledge, attitudes, and practices related to family planning for use in general education and informational programs. Initially the plan was to implement intensive pilot projects in one or two of Taichung City's eleven districts and perhaps in a few villages scattered over the island. The planned pilot programs were escalated to cover the whole city after the rather unexpected success of small-scale pilot action projects and pre-test surveys late in 1961 and early in 1962. The obvious popular demand, as well as the fact that no significant technical or political problems developed in these pilot phases, were the basis for increasing the program's scale. The decision was made in July 1962 to cover all of Taichung in the project and to use a large experimental design which might test a number of important questions.

THE CLASSIC TAICHUNG STUDY

The TPSC surveyed some 2,500 wives ages twenty through thirty-nine in Taichung during October 1962 to January 1963. The subject was knowledge and attitudes toward family planning and actual practice. It was clear from the survey that many women were having more children than they wanted and were trying to do something about it, but not being very successful. It also was found that women were aware of the general decline in infant mortality in Taiwan.

With this background, the Taichung study was planned to answer certain questions about planning and implementing a family planning program.

1. What is the effect of word-of-mouth diffusion of family planning information? From a cost-effectiveness viewpoint, could direct communication to systematically spaced population subgroups affect a much larger population by diffusion?

2. How much can the practice of family planning be increased by a massive information and service campaign of short duration?
3. Do you have to approach both husbands and wives in an educational program, or is it enough to approach the wife alone?
4. Can family planning ideas be spread cheaply and simply by written communication through the mail?
5. What characteristics of couples are most important in determining whether or not they accept family planning methods in the program?
6. What are the characteristics of the many couples who express an intention to accept family planning but fail to do so?
7. Does a new method of contraception, the intrauterine contraceptive device, the Loop, have distinctive advantages in terms of acceptance and diffusion?
8. If there is a significant adoption of family planning, will it accelerate the decline of fertility already begun in Taichung and Taiwan?
9. Was the recent fertility of those accepting family planning high enough so that their use of effective contraception could have produced a distinctively large reduction in birth rates?
10. Which characteristics of couples are related to continuation of effective use of contraception once it is accepted?
11. How did the discussion and perception of what others were doing about family planning affect information and acceptance?

The study's basic design divided the city into comparable sections, each to receive with a different intensity (heavy, medium, light) a different treatment:

1. nothing except posters and some meetings;
2. mailing plus posters and meetings;
3. all major stimuli except a personal visit to the husband; and
4. all stimuli of the program, including a visit to the husband. (See Table 12.)

Table 12. Neighborhood Units (Lins) by Treatment and Density

Treatment	Heavy (13,908)[a]	Medium (11,154)[a]	Light (11,326)[a]	Total (35,388)[a]
Nothing	232	243	292	767
Mail	232	244	292	768
Everything (Wives)	232	122	73	427
Everything (Couples)	232	122	73	427
Total Neighborhood Units	928	731	730	2,389

SOURCE: Berelson and Freedman, *Scientific American, 210:5*, 1964.
[a] Number of women ages 20-39.

In treatments "3" and "4" trained nurse-midwives visited the house. They provided contraceptives at below cost or free, made appointments for wives at local public health service stations, or provided information. The study was designed by Bernard Berelson of the Population Council and Ronald Freedman of the Population Studies Center of the University of Michigan; it was implemented by Dr. J. Y. Peng, then acting director of the Taiwan Maternal and Child Health Institute. The Provincial Maternal and Child Health Institute and the Taiwan Population Studies Center jointly carried out the program from February to October 1963 with the assistance of the Population Council and the Population Studies Center of the University of Michigan. The Taiwan Population Studies Center conducted pre- and post-surveys as the basis for evaluation of the program, and the first effects of the intensive effort were observed through March 31, 1964.

USE OF THE RESULTS

The major findings of the study were as follows.[1]

1. A large information and service campaign of short duration can increase the practice of family planning in a large population of a developing country. (See Table 13.)
2. It may not be necessary to approach both husbands and wives in a family planning program.
3. Home visiting by well-trained fieldworkers was the most effective and efficient educational method.
4. Letters were not effective in increasing the acceptance rate, although the population is fairly literate.
5. Diffusion played a major part in circulating the message, with effects far beyond those on the couples directly influenced by the program.
6. Effective small group meetings had an important role in increasing the acceptance of the IUD.
7. The new intrauterine device was chosen by a large majority of the acceptors.
8. Taichung's fertility decline was accelerated in the year following the experiment, and in 1963-64 exceeded that of the other cities or of the province by a considerable margin.
9. Many families strongly interested in family planning were helped to adopt more satisfactory and effective methods.
10. Such a large-scale effort could be carried out according to plan, with measured results, without political repercussions, and in such a way as to provide a secure basis for the much larger island-wide effort that immediately followed it.

[1] Freedman, R. and J. Y. Takeshita, *Family Planning in Taiwan: An Experiment in Social Change,* Princeton University Press, 1969.

Table 13. Per Cent Contraceptive Acceptance Among Wives 20-39
by Educational Approach

Treatment	Heavy	Medium	Light	Total
Nothing	7	5	5	5
Mail	7	5	6	6
Everything (Wives)	16	13	11	14
Everything (Couples)	18	10	12	15
Total	12	7	7	9

SOURCE: Berelson and Freedman, *Scientific American, 210:5,* 1964.

One of the most important consequences of the Taichung Study was that it set the stage for a renewed effort to bring family planning to the whole island. The Taichung experience showed program administrators that earlier doubts about the readiness of the population were largely unfounded. The overwhelming preference in Taichung City for the new IUD, the Lippes loop, also brought a new method to be the initial focus of the island-wide program. The Taiwanese had had previous IUD experiences with a Japanese device, the Ota ring, used particularly in the cities.

As indicated, an important study finding was that PPH field workers (120 of them existed before the program) were found to be effective in interesting women in IUD insertions, and larger numbers of them were recruited and trained (326 by 1966, including Village Health Education Nurses) for the extended action program to motivate wives — first approaching only those with three or more children and with at least one son. Small group meetings found effective in Taichung were used in some areas and, in a carefully monitored experiment, were found to be more effective per dollar spent than the individual home visits alone. There were problems, however, in training workers to conduct them. The Taichung experiment showed also that a recent birth was an important concomitant to contraceptive acceptance. Building on this finding, the Taiwan program started mailing information with an offer of a free IUD insertion to new mothers shortly after the new baby was registered. This was contrary to the Taichung Study finding that mailing was not effective in motivating women. This finding held back mailing efforts for some time. The inconsistency might have been due to the *timing* of the mailing: postpartum may be a better point to reach a woman with this message. The same was true in the case of the finding of the small difference between visits to both husband and wives and visits to wives only. This finding led the program to concentrate exclusively on reaching wives. Later, the program realized that motivation of the husband is also important because of his role in decision-making. Not much, however, has been made of this approach and in a sense the Taichung Study program has held back program efforts in this regard.

The effectiveness of word-of-mouth diffusion led to use of volunteers from among satisfied users (of the IUD in particular) to facilitate the spread of information.

Based on the finding that even though many acceptors gave up the IUD, not many gave up the idea of contraceptive practice and because of the limited number of workers, the field workers were instructed to visit uncontacted women rather than to follow up the acceptors. They were also instructed to explore new areas rather than to spend time on the old. This had important implications in regard to building up a core of acceptors for a short-term acceptance atmosphere and a long-term result in terms of lack of maintenance for contraceptive continuation.

DOCUMENTATION AND DISSEMINATION

The program activities were recorded carefully and results analyzed and reported quickly through monthly or interim reports and other preliminary reports such as Berelson and Freedman's article in the *Scientific American*, May 1964. This article had extensive circulation in the scientific community and brought early attention from many countries which the Government in Taiwan came to recognize as desirable. In the first general review in English of progress of public health in Taiwan [52], published in 1964, T. C. Hsu, Commissioner of the Taiwan Provincial Health Department, listed "rapid growth of population" as Number 1 of twelve major public health problems in Taiwan. This priority continued for fifteen years and does today. These reports also serve to educate the program staff who produced many documents and reports circulated to their health colleagues in Asia in particular. This benefited other countries which were interested in organizing a family planning program. At the time, the Taichung program was the first large-scale success. It had the glamour of sheer size, and was the only one on which there were data and the success soon became even more wide-scale: the expansion of the Taiwan program (and Korea's) from 1965 onward, for example, helped stimulate programs in the Philippines, Thailand, and Indonesia. Thousands of interested governmental and voluntary agency staff in developing countries were sent to Taiwan for observation under the auspices of USAID, WHO, Ford Foundation, and others promoting family planning. Taiwan began to set up short-term training courses and more arrived. Key figures in the U.S. population and scientific establishment (both university and foundation) were actively involved, and this helped the Taichung study and the program expansion to get considerable circulation internationally. The Population Council, for example, took an active role in disseminating the study results through various publications and informal channels in order to make other countries aware that there had been such a successful trial in Asia.

COMMENTARY

Of particular importance to the effect of this study on the Taiwan program and other countries was the excellent data collection system and the unique organization and approaches to implement program findings.

The study project had an excellent record system for keeping the program directors informed of progress. Activities and acceptances of various contraceptive methods were recorded and reported to the Taiwan Population Studies Center, which analyzed the data quickly to show the results. This rapid feedback system enabled the project directors to make preliminary judgments of the success of the program, and to support a decision — even before the action phase of the experiment was completed — to begin expanding the program to the whole of Taiwan by early 1964. The personnel and resources concentrated in Taichung were shifted to the island-wide program.

Of no small importance, JCRR demanded that action results be shown so that it could get more program funding. This kind of pressure encouraged the program operators to look for the most effective and economical approaches found in the research results and to use them. For the Taichung action program, a medical advisory board composed of eleven leading obstetrics and gynecology specialists (OBGs) in Taiwan was organized. The Board carefully studied the new IUDs and gave its approval for their use in Taichung on a pilot basis. After Taichung, the Board gave its approval for use throughout Taiwan. Because of this involvement of the leading medical authorities, the program was able to train and get the cooperation of private doctors (mostly OBGs) for loop insertions. Of course, the prior experience of these physicians with the Ota ring, another IUD (of Japanese origin), also helped.

The informal organizational set-up of the program had great flexibility. It was part of the Government but yet unofficial. A Committee on Family Health was organized in September 1964 within the Provincial Health Department to implement the island-wide program. It was chaired by the Commissioner of Health. Three of the nine committee members — Commissioner of Health, Chief of the Rural Health Division of JCRR, and the East Asia Representative of the Population Council — formed a standing committee, which met regularly to decide on policy matters and to give technical supervision to the related activities of the voluntary organizations. Under this standing committee, an executive secretary, who was assisted by a three-person working committee, was appointed to carry out the decisions. This committee assumed responsibility only for education and motivation. Actual services were provided by the Maternal and Child Health Association (MCHA), a voluntary organization created in 1964. Because of the lack of a national policy on family planning, this voluntary organization played an important role in implementing those decisions impolitic for the Committee on Family Planning to carry out. The organizational setup with its flexibility, permitted quick change of program direction according to the research findings. This expedited the research results' utilization. (See Figure 13.)

The Taichung experimental project also served as a training ground for TPSC staff, who learned how to operate a program through participation in this study. When the project was found successful, all these personnel were shifted to plan and participate in the island-wide program. The skill and knowledge acquired during the experimental project were transferred .o the larger one without difficulty. Another important factor was that the program directors were all research-oriented and were ~ager to see the research results improve the program. This combination of administrative and applied research experience was unique.

On the other hand, one has to be cautious in claiming Taichung as *the* basis for island-wide program expansion. In some senses the program already had begun with some 120 PPH workers already in place. The particular IUD was an important innovation, of course. Original write-ups of the Taichung Study published internationally were interpreted locally as giving little credit to the persons in Taiwan who had worked diligently both prior to the project to make it possible to execute a study such as Taichung and who worked to carry out the study itself. This oversight complicated a number of programmatic considerations, particularly involving external funding agencies for a decade or more.

SUGGESTIONS FOR DISCUSSION

1. Cuca and Pierce in *Experiments in Family Planning* [30] briefly describe ninety-six experiments in family planning in developing countries. Only twelve of these are classified as "true experiments" in the sense of having both randomization and well-matched control groups. Of these twelve, four were in Taiwan, one being the Taichung Study. What are some of the difficulties in designing studies of this sort in a real-world setting?

2. Certain cultural considerations were important in interpreting the results of this study. For example, findings showed a strong son preference (most couples wanting at least two) and grandmothers (i.e., mother of the husband) clearly had influence over childbearing. These both have to be viewed in the cultural context of Confucianism and familial support systems. How do you make certain that a survey questionnaire incorporates cultural considerations into it? How do you gear into the thinking patterns or cognitive framework of the people whom you wish to learn something from?

3. When an educational intervention takes place seems to have an important bearing on whether it will have an effect. Whether the results of a study will have an effect is also related to timing. How do you relate this concept to the Taichung Study and its impact on an island-wide program expansion?

4. If, as some theories hold, people usually act in their own best interests, what explains why the international agencies in the early and mid 1960s acted so quickly to disseminate the findings of the Taichung Study?

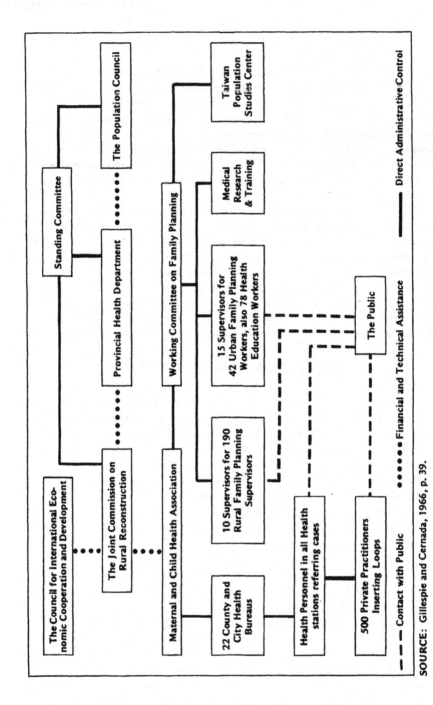

Figure 13. Administrative chart of the family planning program on Taiwan: 1966.

SOURCE: Gillespie and Cernada, 1966, p. 39.

116

6

SUMMARY OF FINDINGS

Case by Case • Cross-Case Analysis

Previous chapters have reviewed factors which facilitated the integration of research findings into program planning, implementation, evaluation and policy development. These have been discussed within the text of each of the eight case studies (Chapter 5). So also have selected organizational, economic, political, cultural, and social barriers to change which existed. Major research utilization and program practice considerations are highlighted in each of the "Commentary" sections within the case studies and also in the "Suggestions for Discussion" section which accompanies each case.

This chapter summarizes major factors facilitating and also hindering research utilization in two ways. It does so first by reviewing findings on a case by case basis and drawing some conclusions. In effect, it gathers together the previous findings in one place and summarizes them. Secondly, the chapter attempts to generalize on the basis of a cross-case analysis, i.e., an elaboration, or synthesis if you will, of common patterns or themes among the many cases presented.

The conclusions drawn from each case may be considered on their own merits and the case by case summary used as a guideline or handy reference. The synthesis of these findings, however, is a bit more than the sum of the parts. It focuses on the Taiwan program as a whole and in its setting. The interaction of the events described in the case studies and of many other such "cases" (as of yet unrecorded) of the Taiwan program's research experience produce a kind of synergetic effect — a dynamic interaction of events which add up to more than the sum of the occurrences themselves. In programmatic terms, it is the *interaction* of these experiences which produced the atmosphere so conducive to effectively applying research to public and program interests, solving problems,

117

and having findings quickly integrated into program activities in the field. To some extent this interaction is considered in the cross-case analysis.

CASE BY CASE

The Case of the Mysteriously Appearing Child

1. All the applied research in the world is not going to solve a practical problem if the persons who must implement the public program are not involved in the early thinking and planning related to proposed research.

2. Both research and program implementation staff need to understand and believe what they are trying to educate the public about. In-service staff education is vital.

3. The communication-persuasion research done in the Western tradition to date offers only minimal guidelines to help choose either informational or educational strategies regarding messages or sources. Application of findings based on such in-school laboratory settings need to be used with caution in the real world.

4. Linkage between governmental agencies at various organizational and hierarchical levels is difficult to achieve. It is possible, however, to locate individuals who because of family ties, social standing, political memberships or even affiliation with a supra-national or international agency may be allowed to provide liaison on an inter-governmental agency level. Such linkage can help bring *useful* research findings to the attention of program implementors and policy makers.

5. There appears to be far more public concern about the expertise and trust-worthiness of provision of services and "educational" output by governmental programs than there is applied research on source credibility. Without this knowledge, some programmatic actions lack direction.

6. In an administrative tug-of-war between research findings and political opposition, "truth" will not always be the predominant factor influencing programmatic output.

7. There is an appropriate and inappropriate time for any educational inter-vention. It is easier to determine the latter. Both researchers and program staff need to be more appreciative of when a program policy maker or chief executive needs to listen to the louder voice of higher-level bureaucrats or the public. Both parties need to keep abreast of just what the political, bureau-cratic and public atmosphere is conducive to in the same manner that they keep posted on research findings or other bureaucratic events.

8. Certain interventions have a symbolic meaning above and beyond their immediate informational impact. The family planning postage stamp is one

which perhaps rises to the level of a clear-cut educational endeavor (i.e., beyond increasing awareness or information) and, indeed, behavioral commitment of vital importance to staff morale and agency and public interpretation of governmental policy.

Sizing Up the Newspapers

1. In-service training where both researchers and program planning and implementation staff can meet in a group discussion setting is useful in getting research used in programs. If a real ongoing program is the subject of such joint discussion, the educational effect is likely to be stronger and the likelihood of research being used greater.

2. Simple marketing types of surveys attempting to answer only one or a few questions make more sense to administrators than more complicated ones, of which Taiwan had its share.

3. One way to get readership response is through a simple offer providing free service or educational materials which either usually cost and/or may be difficult to get otherwise. Cost-effectiveness feedback of this sort, although subject to response bias, is usually easy for an administrator to comprehend and to integrate quickly into his or her plans.

4. Research dealing with the cost-effectiveness of a particular approach is always likely to command the attention of those administrators who hold the program's purse strings.

5. When researchers do not have adequate budgets to carry out needed studies, they sometimes can creatively integrate their objectives with others, as in this mass media experiment piggybacked within a larger one (the Taichung Spacing Incentive Project, described elsewhere in this book).

6. Unanticipated research results, such as the strong male response to the newspaper ad, can sometimes have important program implications. Researchers need to be flexible enough to highlight such findings and present them to program planners in terms of their program applicability. That they were not looking for the results is of no consequence. As the fabled Senator Soaper once said to an agricultural audience, " . . . if it rains during my administration, I take credit for it."

7. The constraints to selecting a particular educational strategy often are interwoven into a complex pattern. Political, budgetary, and bureaucratic restraints held back program development and application of research findings. Some of these restraints were no longer relevant to the present situation, but because they were valid in the past, administrators hesitated venturing into new territory. Researchers need to understand that the perception of the administrator is often as relevant to research utilization as actual program reality. The senior program "historian" is an important resource here.

How Not To Price Oral Contraceptives

1. The degree to which an experiment is generalizable from a limited geographic setting to a larger-scale effort is often determined by two key factors. Well-trained researchers usually are keenly aware of one: the representativeness of the sample being studied. The other is one researchers sometimes forget but administrators cannot: operational validity. This concept involves whether adequate program resources will be available to apply the research and findings. It also deals with the acceptability of the proposed results on a larger-scale. In a sense, this study lacked operational validity for the following reasons:
   a. the program could not afford to dispense oral contraceptives at such a low cost; and
   b. there were serious questions raised about how acceptable the pill was going to be if continuation rates were as low as in the study.

2. Timing is a major obstacle to getting research results applied. If the findings take too long to collect, analyze, and present to administrators, then the program may already have gone ahead to make a major decision regarding the subject studied without waiting for the research findings to be disseminated. Such was the case here.

3. Findings which are not the major focus of the study sometimes may deserve more program application than the major research objectives. In the longer run, the negative attitudes of both fieldworkers and the women of child-bearing age to the oral contraceptives deserved much more attention in terms of program application than the cost-marketing findings.

4. It is possible for health educators to use a simple marketing survey approach to get at the principle of costs. From a methodological viewpoint, the study was most applicable to future program planning. Somehow in the implementation, however, it slowed down and analysis of findings could not keep pace with program action.

Pasting Your Umbrella Before the Rain

1. If large-scale national program action is desired, then research findings need to be translated into a format that program administrators can understand. More importantly in this case, that the public can understand. Synthesizing a variety of research findings into educational objectives and content for a printed booklet requires a working team effort. At a minimum, a linker between researchers and program staff is necessary as well as a skilled interpreter (in this case both writer and editor) to translate for the public. These research utilization "matchmakers" also need to involve the public in the preparation of the product, using as a minimum pretesting and audience response surveys. Under ideal circumstances, this public ought to be collaborators in the development of the product.

2. If various levels of governmental and/or non-governmental agencies must be involved to successfully implement a program based on research findings, then linkage between agencies is essential. Persons functioning within the agencies and partially outside sometimes may serve as linkers. Occasionally foreigners in consultative or resident advisory roles have been used in linker capacities as in this case.

3. If foreign technical assistance is provided either implicitly or explicitly for linkage either between research and applied program action or among various agencies, then a low profile is called for.

4. It often is not possible to isolate and deal with a single dimension or single barrier to getting research utilized. Cultural, bureaucratic and political obstacles to getting knowledge into action are in such a state of dynamic equilibrium that acting upon one often necessarily throws the others out of balance. An accurate diagnosis of the forces restraining or facilitating research utilization is needed much in the same way as the kind of "educational" diagnosis Lewin suggests.

5. No field is more ethnocentric than public health. Sometimes public health agencies (just as individuals) need to practice taking on the role of the other public agencies. Such role-taking may facilitate the understanding of the meaningfulness of survey findings and data to others. Agencies, just as people, usually will act in their own self interest, if they are aware of how such findings can affect them and their relationship with the public.

6. In a practical program, applied research can be useful at many operational stages: in audience surveys to determine public interests, needs, and wants, in pre-testing of materials to fit them more to these needs, and in evaluation of whether these needs are met by the finished product. Both program and research staff need to begin early to share ideas, though, if it is to be accomplished.

7. Knowing that a product or innovation has been tried elsewhere at least identifies the precedent. In reality, however, ethnocentricity sometimes demands that the wheel be re-invented again. A wise original inventor or innovator will forget that he held the patent on the idea and take joy in seeing others assimilate the innovation as their very own idea.

Free Offers For a Limited Time Only

1. Paying close attention to feedback from consumers of service and home-visiting field workers is a must if applied research is to be able to focus on ongoing program needs *when* they are current. To collect this kind of data an organizational framework is needed which systematically feeds information back from the field to both program headquarters and research and evaluation staff and back again to the field.

2. A great deal of flexibility is needed to conduct operations research. Program and research staff need to work together closely. Applied researchers need to be able to act upon data from service statistics, consumer surveys, and observations of field and supervisory staff. With this flexibility to shift the research focus to try new approaches or variations on old ones, researchers can meet program needs *when* they develop.

3. Some measure of faith by both research and program staff is necessary occasionally. Knowing that an operations research-oriented innovative project works does not always mean that anyone knows exactly why it works. Whether this particular project facilitated decision-making because of its "limited time" offer or whether its very availability stimulated greater worker input, or both, is as yet unknown. Separating the effects of these two considerations was never quite possible in the field.

4. To achieve rapid wider scale expansion of single operations research projects, it is essential (in addition to many other considerations) to have a built-in evaluative device. The excellent feedback system of service statistics about contraceptive acceptors and their socio-demographic characteristics enabled the field workers, their supervisors, and both the program and research staff at headquarters, to see the project results quickly. This enabled rapid expansion and project variations on a wider-scale throughout the Island.

5. Applied research done at the request of field staff and in line with consumer interests to meet program needs workers identify has high potential for being utilized if it can produce visible results.

Today Kaohsiung, Tomorrow Taiwan

1. Communication-oriented operations research carried out and designed collaboratively by both researchers and program planners who are based in a single organizational unit can have its results applied in action programs rapidly. This finding runs against a general trend, presumably to increase the "objectivity" of evaluation, to separate research and evaluation from program units.

2. Quick feedback of research findings to administrators, geared to their own frames of reference (i.e., related to consistency with government policy, non-threatening, and within budgetary limitations), and in ways easily translated to action (i.e., self-explanatory tables, graphs, charts, etc.) help get results integrated in program action.

3. Research results dealing with behavioral change need highlighting for these are usually more useful criteria for administrators taking program action than changes in awareness, knowledge or attitude. For family planning programs, fertility declines are an even better criterion, if less likely to be demonstrable at least over the short run.

4. It is important to use research findings not only to implement programs but also to integrate methodologies into other ongoing research. For example, the Kaohsiung mass media survey inventories were integrated into annual Island-wide surveys to collect information on a regular basis and integrate it into national-level program plans.

5. Administrators seem especially impressed by research findings that the population they are part of differs significantly from others. For example, the cultural finding that many women viewed weight gain as an advantage rather than an undesirable side effect. This finding was one likely to be integrated into program action if only because it was so clearly non-Western.

6. A lack of experience with an approach, mass media in this case, can be a major handicap to program adoption. A pilot or demonstration study can help overcome this handicap and also produce a corps of experienced staff for future program action.

Incentives: Beyond Family Planning

1. It is an advantage to a governmental agency to set up a controversial experimental research project through a voluntary agency. There is a disadvantage, however, in that at some point the government planners may need to provide this child their name. To bring this about, there has to be a phasing-into process integrated into the plan in order to achieve the transition.

2. Longer-term but smaller-scale research projects which are designed to be expanded on a larger scale (if successful) need to involve long-term social and economic planners. Considerations of inflation and cultural interactions must be built into planning. Both the Year of the Dragon and changes in female employment caused unanticipated cultural problems here.

3. Sometimes unusually innovative research which has a minimal potential for expansion on a large scale in the country it is conducted in may find its results more usable in other countries. In some cases, the doing of the research may be based upon larger political goals relating to maintaining a leadership position among other countries carrying out similar social programs. In Taiwan, such was an important consideration.

4. Applied research projects may have more chance of being accepted as research and/or their findings applied in programs if they build upon previously-existing similar projects (e.g., incentives).

5. A research project which would have to be implemented by agencies other than the one(s) carrying out the research needs to build in ways to involve these other agencies. Linkage with agencies at higher governmental levels (e.g., advisory committees) may be necessary to expand a program on a wider or national scale. When research findings show successful results which have

potential for replicability, it may help to allow the higher-level agency leaders to take credit for the project after the fact.

Scientific American Goes Asian

1. An organizational structure which has considerable flexibility can more easily implement research which is directed toward program action. This flexibility can, among other things, help avoid political repercussions (as in the case of certain functions being carried on by a "semi-voluntary" agency) and expedite rapid changing of program directions based on preliminary research findings.

2. The extent to which research findings get utilized can depend to some extent upon the magnitude of the research project. Large-scale findings drawn from a project which has the virtue of sheer size (e.g., Taichung) can be impressive to administrators both at home and abroad.

3. The utility of research also can be related to the success of a "first." The novelty of a major breakthrough in innovation testing can, of itself, be a virtue which does not go unnoticed by upwardly mobile administrators wishing to associate themselves with a recognized success.

4. Having strong international organization inputs on a research project can have an interesting diffusion effect. Sometimes international publicity about a national project extends to many other countries. Eventually it finds its way back to the country of origin in the form of international praise. Such praise under certain political circumstances can be a considerable stimulus to adopt research findings in program activities at the national level which might otherwise be slower in occurring.

5. Having a corps of administrators who have had strong working relationships with researchers and who have had previous experience adapting findings to programs can make the process much easier.

6. Rapid feedback of results from ongoing applied research (and a system developed for this purpose) is necessary, in order not to miss the possibilities for integrating findings into an expanding program. If feedback is too slow, the opportunity is lost.

CROSS-CASE ANALYSIS

Certain common patterns may be noted among the cases and the summary of findings presented above. Some have been noted earlier in Chapter Four's analysis of selected factors favorable to family planning research utilization. Together, these common themes interacted historically to produce the atmosphere in Taiwan which was so conducive to getting research results integrated into an ongoing family planning program. A brief analysis of the findings is presented here on a cross-case basis. This synthesis is followed in Chapter 7 by a review of some of the implications for general health education practice and development of a stronger theoretical base.

Political Purpose

The Government had a long-time policy of providing technical assistance to less economically developed countries. Agricultural development and land reform were two major areas of aid. Family planning became the third. Thusly, the program although organizationally placed within the Health Department, which was at a low level in the governmental bureaucratic hierarchy, actually had a higher political priority. Taiwan felt it needed to maintain a close relationship with the United States and to continue its membership in the United Nations representing China. Such technical assistance programs enhanced its international image. When the President of the World Bank, Robert McNamara, decided to stop in Taiwan in 1970, for example, it was to fly into Taichung to visit the family planning program which had become a model for all of Asia. The political value of the program was never lost on national leaders, particularly economic planners who were strong backers of the effort. Such political backing meant that funds and resources were made available to attract skilled researchers and program implementors who also recognized the value of being in the international spotlight. They in turn were ready to take risks, to experiment, to try new approaches to better the previous ones.

Readiness to Change

Taiwan was undergoing a kind of economic revolution. It was being cited throughout the Western world and Asia as a model of sound economic development. People's ways of life were changing as per capita income rose sharply and they took part in an unusually equitable system of distribution of income. There was a readiness for change, an adoption of new ideas, whether it was agricultural — hybrid strains of rice, intensive fertilization — or clothing — synthetic fibers, new dyes, western styles. This general atmosphere of change manifested itself even in governmental agencies, particularly newer ones such as those conducting the family planning program. And it inevitably manifested itself in an open attitude toward trying new ways to improve programs. Methodological approaches and scientific knowledge were harnessed to strengthen applied research and use findings to provide better service.

Research Purpose

There was little doubt from the beginning of the program what the function of the research component was to be. Research was intended to improve the program, to broaden its scope, and to plan future operations which would meet potential consumer wants and needs. The focus was *applied research*. It included field experiments, pilot projects, operations research, social surveys, field observation and data feedback systems. It was tied in closely with the ongoing evaluation built into many program operations. Cost-effectiveness studies played an important role at the early stages when funding was limited. Theoretical and methodological approaches were selected to fit the action program problem, rather than the more common opposite.

Centralized Organization

Both the research and the action program units were for the most part the responsibility of a single agency under one directorship and housed under a single roof. Although much is said by public health experts and armchair observers about the need to separate certain evaluative and most research functions from ongoing programmatic ones, more needs to be said in defense of combining such units organizationally. In such an atmosphere, researchers learn how to gear into the interests and thinking patterns of administrators and administrators learn about the researchers. *Proximity* increases the potential for joint planning at early stages of program and research activities. It also decreases the time needed to get research results translated into operational terms and, thusly, increases the likelihood of utilizing these results.

Linkage

The family planning program had its strongest backing from economic planners, particularly, Minister Without Portfolio, K. T. Li, a former Minister of Economic Affairs and also of Finance. Various high-level officials in many Ministries were strong backers. One of the strongest linking agencies among these various hierarchical levels was the Sino-American Joint Commission on Rural Construction. The director of its Rural Health Division, Dr. S. C. Hsu, liased frequently among political party officials, governmental administrators, legislators, voluntary agency staff, etc. Within the confines of the family planning organization, resident foreign advisors were used to help translate research findings into implementable programmatic actions.

Systematic Feedback

There was an unusually comprehensive two-way flow of communication between the field and headquarters: service statistics, input-output indices, regular headquarters staff meetings, field staff meetings, meetings of field and headquarters staff. The field workers often were the first to learn from people in the villages what was right or wrong in the program. Social surveys were conducted on a regular basis to assess changes in public knowledge, attitudes and behavior, to determine the nature of contraceptive side-effects and to deal with them. Extensive documentation also was carried out as was dissemination of information.

Other-Orientation

A major focus of in-service education was to help staff from the evaluation/ research units and those from the program implementation units learn how each defined given situations. Training sessions brought staff from both areas together to plan ongoing programs and discuss the pros and cons of their contributions. They were encouraged to take on the role of the other in discussion. This interaction helped develop trust and also an understanding of the interdependency of staff functions.

Where less success was evident was in agencies learning to take on the role of the other. Few fields are more ethnocentric than public health and Taiwan was no exception. The inability of public health to gear into the needs of other fields such as education (i.e., formal) was a serious handicap for much less was done to educate the educators about population research implications than was possible.

Operational Validity

If a research project deals with an innovation which cannot be operationalized it is going to be a wasted effort. Some of Taiwan's success in utilizing its research findings certainly has to be attributed to its adherence to two fundamental components of what may be termed operational validity. These consist of being certain that adequate program resources (funds, know-how, staff) can be available to implement a project and that the potential implementation has some likelihood of public acceptability.

Competition and Collaboration

Taiwan monitored carefully the results of ongoing family planning programs in other countries, particularly Asian. Visits back and forth to other countries by program and research staff were frequent in the late 1960's and early 1970's. Through international agencies such as the Population Council and from national ministries Taiwan staff often had monthly reports available. A considerable competition developed between Taiwan and South Korea to provide contraception to greater percentages of married couples of child-bearing ages. This was also true in lesser ways with Hong Kong and Singapore and later Thailand. To some extent this increased the readiness of both Taiwan and Korea to experiment with new ways of reaching the public and of quickly implementing findings of studies. These various exchanges also brought about collaborative efforts between the two countries to share research and program findings. In the 1970's the International Committee for Applied Research on Population (ICARP) was formally developed with Population Council technical assistance to share and disseminate evaluation and research findings on a regional basis (Taiwan worked closely with the Korean, Bangladesh, Thailand, Philippine, and Indonesian programs).

Synergy

The whole is equal to more than the sum of its parts. An inventory of some of the parts, however, is needed to determine what the whole was. The parts included political purpose, readiness to change, an applied research focus, centralized organization, linkage, systematic feedback, an other-orientation, operational validity and competition/collaboration considerations, as mentioned earlier. They also included, as noted in Chapter 4, an incentive or reward system, an atmosphere of trust, an unusual documentation and dissemination system, flexibility to adapt research while it was ongoing, rapid feedback of results, and a talent for building on accumulated experience. It was with the dynamic interaction of these variables that the program was able in any given instance to bridge the gap between research and program operations and to consistently do it successfully.

7

COMMUNITY HEALTH
EDUCATION IMPLICATIONS

Overview • Improving Practice •
Toward a Stronger Theoretical Base

OVERVIEW

Much of what has been said previously deals with getting research findings used in an ongoing family planning program. Certain factors discussed obviously are of considerable concern to working community health educators — both in family planning or any other socio-health-oriented programs, whether in the so-called "developing" or "developed" countries.

The author of a book on this topic cannot excuse himself from the obligation to his readers of translating his own research findings into some guidelines for practical program use. He hopes that in Chapter 5, the reader will find the "Commentary" and "Questions for Discussion" section useful in understanding the program implications of each study. These and the summary of findings (analyzed on a case by case basis and also cross-case) in Chapter 6 should be useful guidelines for those involved in conducting research or applying it to programs. Certainly community health educators will be among those who might profit from the reading. This Chapter, however, attempts to reinforce some conclusions and address them specifically to the broad area of community health education programs, both in terms of practice and of developing a stronger theoretical base.

IMPROVING PRACTICE

A major problem in the field in the United States today is less how to get research results utilized in programs than how to get more competent researchers. With the exception of some infrequent basic research by associated behavioral scientists, most research done by community health educators should be applied. Such is the nature of the job description. Unfortunately, this health education research too often is carried out by persons with inadequate theoretical or methodological training. Thus, prospects for application are limited for the studies are badly designed, poorly executed, and inadequately analyzed. A major concern for the profession is how to attract and train more persons to our professional schools, particularly doctoral programs at Schools of Public Health, to carry out this applied research. The numbers of graduates of such programs are presently not sufficient even to fill faculty vacancies at the Schools themselves, let alone agency settings. If the research arm of the profession is not to become extinct in the next decade, then there needs to be an intensive effort to recruit and train these individuals. Otherwise, community health education research is going to be relegated to school health and exercise science studies and the remainder of the field dabbled in by medical sociologists, medical anthropologists and others more concerned with social interaction than user/ consumer orientations. If we could channel a tenth of the professional effort we now are devoting to professional role delineation and the mating of such improbable bedfellows as school and community health educators, there might be hope that some of us will not meet the fate of the dinosaur — or the *auk,* who as Ogden Nash noted, became "extinct because he forgot how to fly, and could only *walk.*"[1]

Beyond developing a corps of well-trained applied researchers, the field of community health education badly needs to draw together and codify its theoretical orientations. With such conceptual notions assembled and available easily, field practitioners would be able to "anticipate solutions" and have "greater insight into explanations of why things turned out as they did." This suggestion, made by Dorothy Nyswander [53] some twenty-five years ago, has yet to be implemented. Some of us need to take action soon or all there will be for the health educator emeritus to look back to a quarter of a century from now will be a collection of outdated and stereotypic maxims. There have to be more meaningful epitaphs than "Start Where The People Are" or "Learn By Doing."

[1] From "A Caution to Everybody," *The New Pocket Anthology of American Verse* (ed. Oscar Williams), Pocket Books Inc., New York, p. 346, 1955.

TOWARD A STRONGER THEORETICAL BASE

As Lewin has said, there is nothing more practical than a good theory [54]. This slender volume hardly purports to present a new theory of research utilization. It does, however, identify and analyze some research utilization principles which have been tested in the field and provide some synthesis. Underlying these findings are certain theoretical orientations and concepts which seem to have applicability beyond the area of research utilization. A summary of a half dozen of these underlying theoretical orientations which appear to have broader application to community health education and which are not getting the attention they deserve in our field follows.

Mass Communications

One relevant statement (mine) of the historical evolvement of mass communication theory or typologies has been from Lasswell's [55]

> WHO
> SAYS WHAT
> IN WHICH CHANNEL
> TO WHOM
> WITH WHAT EFFECT?

to Berelson's [56] recognition that the theory of all-powerful mass media had been challenged:

> SOME KINDS OF COMMUNICATION
> ON SOME KINDS OF ISSUES
> BROUGHT TO THE ATTENTION OF SOME KINDS OF
>   PEOPLE
> UNDER SOME KINDS OF CONDITIONS
> HAVE SOME KINDS OF EFFECTS.

In addition to this recognition of the interaction of social factors and individual differences, a newer set of propositions or principles incorporating the perspective of the receiver or user of communications as an active manager of information has been proposed [57]. Essentially, this third orientation inverts the usual pyramid which finds the source or sender of the message, or the "communication" as key focal points and concentrates on the more active role of the consumer or user. Thusly, from this third statement, "target" audiences and "passive recipients" of messages are not likely to be guidelines for sound community health education planning in the area of communications. As Cernada has stated,

> WHO SELECTS WHAT COMMUNICATIONS
> ON ANY ISSUES

ONLY FROM *WHOM* THEY WISH
AND ONLY THROUGH THE *CHANNEL* THEY SELECT
AND WHATEVER *EFFECT* THERE IS
DEPENDS UPON WHO'S *INTERPRETATION* OF THE
PLACE OF THAT MESSAGE, THAT SOURCE, THAT
CHANNEL IN THEIR *OWN REAL WORLD.*

The theoretical orientation of the typology presented above is based on a fusion of communication theory with underlying concepts drawn from symbolic interactionism. If the practicing community health educator or applied researcher adopts this kind of user-focused orientation, he or she is not only in step with traditional health education principles (e.g., as espoused by Nyswander [53]) but also will see the value of balancing more traditional deductive methods of investigating health education problems with more inductive methodologies (e.g., participant observation and interviews). As Mullen and Reynolds [58] indicate in their both theoretically and practically useful discussion of the implications of Grounded Theory for linking health education practice and theory, such approaches lessen the likelihood of programs and research engaging in blaming the victim.

The Problem-Solver Perspective

This theoretical model flows from the work of Watson [59], Lippitt [60], Miles [61], Jung [62], and others. Havelock [5] (see Chapter 2) cites it as being one of three related to research utilization (in addition to the Research, Development and Diffusion model and the Social Interaction model) and attempts to fuse these three into his own variation. The Problem-Solver (PS) perspective is one that deserves more attention in terms of community health education programming as well as research. It lessens the likelihood that we will "blame the victim" as well as provides a useful framework to apply methodologies which move us beyond lip service to the old maxim, "Start Where The People Are." This more holistic, consumer-oriented model of communication posits that:[2]

- AN EDUCATIONAL DIAGNOSIS OF THE SITUATION OUGHT TO BE MADE BY THE POTENTIAL USER SINCE THIS IS AN EDUCATIONALLY SOUND GIVEN OF LEARNING THEORY;
- THUSLY, THE NEEDS OF THE USER ARE THE CHANGE AGENT'S MAJOR CONCERN;
- THE CHANGE AGENT IS A CATALYST OR CONSULTANT OR COLLABORATOR, NOT A MANIPULATOR;

---

[2] The above are adapted from Havelock [5] and modified by the author to CHE practice.

- THE CHANGE AGENT'S JOB IS TO HELP THE USER TAKE ADVANTAGE OF HIS/HER INTERNAL RESOURCES; and
- SELF-INITIATED CHANGE HAS THE FIRMEST MOTIVATIONAL BASIS AND BEST PROSPECTS FOR LONG-TERM MAINTENANCE.

Perception

- START WHERE PEOPLE ARE (OUTDATED MAXIM OF UNKNOWN ORIGIN);
- THE PERCEPTIONS OF THOSE WHO ARE TO BE TAUGHT FURNISH IMPORTANT DATA TO BE USED IN PROGRAM PLANNING (NYSWANDER, 1956) [53]; and
- THE ALERT HEALTH WORKER . . . MUST DEVELOP SKILL AS AN OCULIST, TRAINING HIMSELF TO LOOK AT HIS SPECTACLES AND NOT MERELY THROUGH THEM, AND TRAINING HIMSELF TO LOOK BOTH AT AND THROUGH THE SPECTACLES OF THE CLIENT WITH WHOM HE DEALS (ALLPORT, 1958) [63].

Some more recent perspectives of perception which also have a place in community health education are:

- A'S PERCEPTION OF B IS INFLUENCED NOT ONLY BY A'S GENERAL OR SPECIFIC PERSPECTIVE OF B BUT ALSO BY A'S PERCEPTION OF B'S PERCEPTION OF A. B'S PERCEPTION OF A IS INFLUENCED NOT ONLY BY B'S GENERAL OR SPECIFIC PERSPECTIVE OF A BUT ALSO BY B'S PERCEPTION OF A'S PERCEPTION OF B. THEY BOTH, IN TURN, ARE INFLUENCED BY THEIR PERCEPTION OF THE OTHER'S INTERPRETATION OF THE SITUATION AT HAND. (Recent thinking on Face to Face Interaction which can become more complicated as A and B become more sophisticated in interpreting the other's perception).
- PERCEPTION CANNOT BE EMPHASIZED TO THE DETRIMENT OF ENVIRONMENT OR WE CAN BECOME PERCEPTIVE VICTIM BLAMERS (CERNADA, 1943).[3]

The Change Continuum

The presumption that attitude change must precede behavioral change is a theoretical assumption integrated into practice by health education from social psychology long ago. Briefly stated, it defines the relation of attitude to

---

[3] This principle was based upon the author's early experience in an unheated classroom in Somerville Massachusetts, circa 1943 after the teacher had recommended that the students think "warm." It was suggested that the boiler's breakdown was related to the students' pronounced tendency to not take morning prayers seriously.

behavior in terms of an attitude change/behavioral change sequence. If behavior is to change, the way to bring it about is to work on attitude change:

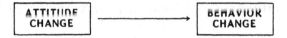

Within the field of social psychology, this theoretical assumption has been challenged in a variety of ways. M. Brewster Smith [64] has tried to counter this tendency to exaggerate the causal importance of attitudes (or even situations) alone by emphasizing other variables affecting behavior such as distal social antecedents (historic conditions), socio-cultural environment and personality. Others in social psychology have stressed the need to consider dimensions within the attitude sphere, e.g., the affective, cognitive and behavioral intent components, intensity, salience, importance, social constraints, inter-relationships with other attitudes and beliefs, and situational variables. In summary, the attitude toward attitude has changed elsewhere and community health educators need to be attuned to the implications for practice.

If it is so, as some theorists (e.g., those of the Cognitive Dissonance orientation) postulate, that induced behavioral change brings about attitude change, then the implications for health education are many. This model of change becomes:

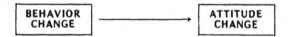

Furthermore, if as supposed [65], structural or environmental changes (e.g., legislation, working procedures, job content, interaction patterns) can bring about behavior changes which are followed by attitude changes (job satisfaction, empathy), then a logical pattern for community health education intervention strategy selection may be:

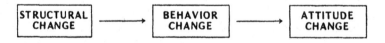

Trainers and organizational development specialists have used this approach extensively but in closed settings. Group dynamics espouses similar change concepts but in small group settings. Large-scale application has potential for expansion. Although such a change strategy may seem the longest way to get from one point to the other, it may sometimes be the shortest distance in terms of achieving change and possibly of maintaining it.

Other-Orientation

Two major drawbacks to effective public health and social development programs are *egocentrism* and *ethnocentrism* (the group counterpart of egocentrism). These manifest themselves in our natural tendency as change agents to be more concerned with what we want than what the individual or community we serve wants. Examples abound: the U.S. university carrying out research to suit faculty interests rather than program needs; the pater-familias and advocacy roles of change agents which assume they know best what is in the public interest and how best to provide it; agencies projecting their own ethnocentric customs and established ways of doing things on people who have different ways based on different past learning experiences. As Goodenough suggests of community development programs, an *other-orientation* is needed. This orientation enable us to shed our ego and ethnocentric views and identify and empathize more with others, "see the world from *their* point of view." [66]

One underlying orientation of the "other-oriented" view is Symbolic Interaction Theory. This theory supposes that meanings are constructed from social interaction in which a person sizes up a situation, weighs factors relevant to him or her and takes action accordingly. To influence another person's behavior, the change agent needs to understand the person's perspective, i.e., the meaning a particular behavior has for her, how she organizes her knowledge of the world, and how she goes about deciding what action to take. Any educational intervention by the change agent must address how the person defines the particular situation of concern. This *definition of the situation* is that person's categorization of just what a particular event means in his or her own real world. Not what it means to the change agent or what the change agent supposes it to mean based on inadequate attention to the person of concern. Change agents need to be trained in and practice more frequently techniques of *gearing into* and taking on the *role of the other*. Those involve learning about what another person views as matters of concern to him or her and how these interact in his or her own real (or phenomenological) world. They also involve developing empathy so that one can better understand what a particular event means to this person. Carrying out these functions effectively requires training in information gathering, comparison of information from various sources, openness, reality testing, and risk-taking. The outcome is to reduce some of the social distance between the change agent and the user and enable the change agent to be able to communicate and work in this other person's world.

Learning Theory

A major underpinning of health education is learning theory. Too often health educators neglect some of the more basic principles of the kind of learning process we become involved in. Nyswander [53] alerts us to such significant learning opportunities as involving people in the planning process for it is an educational method of itself to bring about change, of using the program evaluation process as an educational method for staff, of the interaction of group and task in most processes, and of community organization to bring about change. We, unfortunately, do not always take advantage of such opportunities for we are too often concerned with short-term educational and program objectives. We tend to neglect the longer-term objectives of education, e.g., at national development levels, where a major function of education can be to create *self-reliance* (Nyerere) [67] or at the individual or communal level where education can provide people with the power to control their own lives (Friere) [68].

Some rather simplistic but pertinent educational principles (or perhaps only maxims) by Pine and Horn [69] which are worth being printed on all health educators' union cards (one hesitates to advocate tatoos if only for aesthetic reasons), follows:

- Learning is an experience which occurs inside the learner and is activated by the learner.
- No one directly teaches anyone anything of significance.
- Learning is the discovery of the personal meaning and relevance of ideas.
- Learning (behavioral change) is a consequence of experience.
- Learning is a cooperative and collaborative process.
- Learning is an evolutionary process.
- Learning is sometimes a painful process.
- One of the richest resources for learning is the learner himself.
- The process of learning is emotional as well as intellectual.
- The processes of problem solving and learning are highly unique and individual.

Lion's Head, Snake's Tail: A Conclusion

The reader about here will remember that the purpose of this slender volume was not to catalogue the substantial body of social and behavioral science theory on which community health education is based. The half-dozen theoretical concepts presented here were chosen because their interaction seems to this writer to be the basis for a way of approaching planned social change. They also are dealt with because they flow from the case study (although not without imaginative priming) and because they illustrate Lewin's notion that there is nothing more practical than a good theory. The need to gather together and codify the underlying theoretical orientations of community health education remains.

APPENDIX

A

EWCI RECOMMENDATIONS FOR RESEARCH UTILIZATION

*Summary of recommendations from the
East-West Communication Institute's Conference on
"Making Population —Family Planning Research
Useful: The Communicator's Contribution." [2]*

EWCI CONFERENCE RECOMMENDATIONS

From Research Group

1. Research utilization should be directed to operational officers in population programs as well as directed to administrators.

2. Research and development activities should be encouraged outside of family planning agencies as well as in the research units of family planning agencies.

3. While it is probably unwise to assume that most administrators know what research should be done, program administrators are able to enumerate what problems they have. The problems enumerated by administrators should be translated into high priority concerns for research.

4. Developing country research agencies should be encouraged to accept the research methods developed in Western social science but not necessarily the variables and previous substantive results of Western social science. The research methods adopted should include survey research, experimental designs, participant observation, and the full range of data collection and analysis methodologies.

5. Administrators should educate funding agencies and legislative supporters to the facts that:
   a) research is necessary to evaluate new programs and funds must be allocated for research; and

b) the research results may show negative evaluations of current programs without indicating that the administrators have poorly carried out their responsibilities.

6. More than quantitative demographic research is required to make research useful to administrators and others.

7. Summaries of successful research applications should be prepared and disseminated to program administrators. These summaries should be case studies that show where and how research results have been applied to modify programs and increase their success.

8. Transnational research studies should pay particular attention to cultural variables in addition to variables which are useful cross-nationally. National needs are more important than cross-national comparability.

9. Administrators should recognize that research cannot provide all the answers. Research results are only one input into policy decision-making.

10. A recognition system (salary, prestige, etc.) should be established for researchers who make their research utilizable and participate in its utilization.

11. All research proposals should include a section stating the potential applicability of the research. Part of the contract should include funds for publication and dissemination by personal contacts with administrators and operational officers. Donor agencies should also support publications such as information materials for appropriate audiences and journals for professional associations.

12. Donor agencies should provide small grants to facilitate the development of professional associations for disciplines related to population.

13. Funds should be provided in all countries for the selection and synthesis of research results as well as conducting original research.

14. Researchers should be provided with access to communication support services. Communicators should be provided access to researchers to assess the accuracy of what they communicate.

15. Applied population research training should be supported in every country. The long-term development of sufficiently trained manpower is mandatory.

16. More attention should be given to the ethical implications of information campaigns and other population communication efforts.

17. Research colonialism should be discouraged.

18. Every research project should allocate funds to increase the pool of trained manpower as well as conducting the research itself.

19. More research funds should be allocated to:
a) studies of the management and organization of family planning programs;

    b) studies of motivational and communication aspects of demographic behavior and policies; and

    c) studies of the relationship of family planning programs to the overall development plans and strategies of every country.

20. Female researchers are discriminated against in population research and should not be. Discrimination is particularly evident in the international donor agencies. More females should be involved in the research and administration of population programs, in the population divisions of international donor agencies (particularly in responsible field advisory positions), and in research on the development of contraceptive methods. It must be recognized that women can often make contributions because they are women and not only because they are equal.

21. More young researchers should be involved in responsible research positions. Further, ethnic representativeness among researchers should be encouraged in countries where this condition does not already exist.

22. In order to influence the allocation of research funds, the Boards of Family Planning Agencies and International Donor Agencies should include representatives of the consumers of their services and funds.

From the Linker Group

1. Although there is need for some mechanism and procedure to bridge the gap between research results and their use in programs, it should not be thought of as an individual or institutional role such as "linker," "middleman," "processor," "transducer," etc., but as *a process in which the essential element is a relationship* between those who need to know with those who are in a position to help them find out. The process begins at the point when a research question is identified and continues through the use of findings in programs including feedback to researchers of problems related to application.

2. Important in the development of relationships is the recognition of the multiple roles which may be played by *researchers* and *users* and those who help to *link* them. Results of research and of application of research must be disseminated selectively to each of these groups.

3. In recognition of the importance of the relationships involved, thought should be given to *short courses and conferences* where research, findings in specific subject areas would be communicated. The form and format should be selected depending on the audience — for example, for a group of political leaders, research results might best be processed into film while administrators might be perfectly comfortable with printed reports including adequate graphs, charts, and other illustrations.

4. Funds should be made available for selectively inserting important research-based information into meetings, conferences, and training programs. These should also serve as opportunities for feedback from such specialized user groups.

5. *Information analysis centers* embodying documentation, library and information resources are needed at national, regional, and international levels. There should be networking of such facilities at all levels to insure two-way flow of research results and resulting technical information. Information analysis centers should be adequately funded to perform the full range of identifying, collecting, classifying, processing, retrieving, and disseminating information in usable form to specific users in practical time frames.

6. Emphasis should be on improving the information system as it exists in the countries, stressing exchange of research based information within each country as well as internationally.

7. In order to enhance the country networks, action should be taken to identify the entry points in the information system, find out who the key access people are, and provide them training to better use the system. If the entry points are *in* only, then parallel *out* points should be developed.

8. Basic elements in the *country network* should be the teaching, training, research, and other educational institutions, since they provide the element of relationship between researchers and users essential to effective research utilization.

9. Recognizing that the development of sophisticated national, regional, and international networks will be a long-term process, thought should be given to utilizing existing country teaching and training institutions as important means of getting research results to relevant users.

From the Research Users Group
(Administrators, Operational Officers, and Others)

1. Collecting, consolidating, storing, processing, and disseminating the existing body of knowledge in each country should be undertaken by *a national institution*. This institution should maintain a continuous link with all other relevant national agencies producing and using research and with relevant agencies.

2. Responsibility for program-originated research should be given to *a research manager* who would insure that research is tailored to the program. The research manager should diagnose program problems, identify research needs, feed readily available information into research, initiate and promote needed research utilizing national capacities. He should communicate

available research findings to administrators on terms of program implications. He should feed researchers problems for investigation which grow out of attempts to apply results. He should provide information to other components of the family planning program and related programs. Less international influence should be exercised on the initiation of research projects.

3. *More funds* should be allocated to studies of management and organization of family planning programs, studies of motivation and communication, demographic behavior and policy and relationship of the family and population program to the overall development plan and strategy.

APPENDIX
B

PRELIMINARY ANALYSIS OF MASS MEDIA: 1966–1970

An internal memo to program administrators suggesting choices of mass media methods based on findings of three Island-wide sample surveys.

Herewith are some suggestions about choice of mass media methods, based primarily on the latest findings of the third Island-wide KAP Survey (1970), but in selected instances also on the Economic Correlates Survey (of Husbands, 1969) and the Kaohsiung Surveys (1966 and 1968). These are preliminary and done in haste and should be the subject of further analysis and discussion with the concerned program staff. The outcome might be that you mimeograph this or a revised version for staff reference in planning future mass media expenditures.

The major deviation I see from our present approach is that more attention needs to be paid to making content of messages as specific as possible, trying to get more TV time, eliminating *Harvest* magazine, and trying to work out special arrangements with the *United Daily* and *China Time* newspapers.

POINT 1: THE VALUE

It is worth using mass media due to the large audience. For further details, refer to Table B-1.

POINT 2: CONTENT

It is clear from the findings of KAP III (1970) that all public information should do more than just mention a contraceptive method. It is not

* G. Cernada, The Population Council, July 30, 1970.

Table B-1. Taiwan's Mass Media Audience

Those Who:	Economics (1969) Husbands (Per Cent)	KAP III (1970) Wives (Per Cent)	Kaohsiung (1966) Wives (Per Cent)
Listen to *RADIO*	64	60	62
Watch *TV*	43	59	25
Read *NEWSPAPERS*	58	30	29
Go to *MOVIES*	63	48	48
Read *MAGAZINES*	24	15	19
Listen to radio *daily*	23	18	49
Watch TV *daily*	18	27	11
Read newspapers *daily*	38	15	18
Go to movies *once/month or more*	33	14	32
Read magazines *sometimes/often*	24	15	16

Table B-2. Per Cent Wives Knowing About Loop and Pill

	Knowledge Of:	
	Loop (Per Cent)	Pill (Per Cent)
Did not know of method	20	30
Knew of but did not know how to use it	24	35
Knew how to use but never used it	30	25
Knew and never used	26	10

enough to know of the method. P. I. ought to tell how it is used, where to get it, its advantages, and how much it costs, etc. Motivational and *small family* materials should go only to young people and be only a small part of the total output. (See Table B-2.)

POINT 3: SELECTIVITY

There clearly are favorite programs and subjects which, if selected, will reach larger numbers of wives according to the KAP III Survey. (See Tables B-3, B-4, B-5, and B-6.)

Table B-3. Favorites: Radio

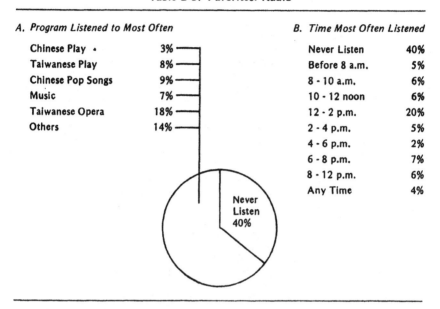

A. *Program Listened to Most Often*

Chinese Play •	3%
Taiwanese Play	8%
Chinese Pop Songs	9%
Music	7%
Taiwanese Opera	18%
Others	14%

B. *Time Most Often Listened*

Never Listen	40%
Before 8 a.m.	5%
8 - 10 a.m.	6%
10 - 12 noon	6%
12 - 2 p.m.	20%
2 - 4 p.m.	5%
4 - 6 p.m.	2%
6 - 8 p.m.	7%
8 - 12 p.m.	6%
Any Time	4%

Never Listen 40%

Table B-4. Favorites: TV

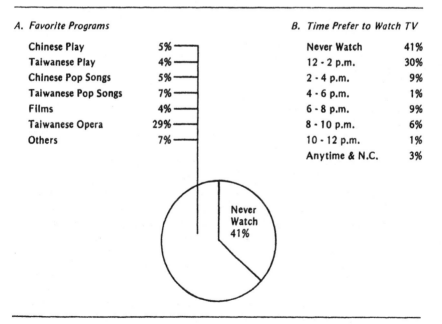

A. *Favorite Programs*

Chinese Play	5%
Taiwanese Play	4%
Chinese Pop Songs	5%
Taiwanese Pop Songs	7%
Films	4%
Taiwanese Opera	29%
Others	7%

B. *Time Prefer to Watch TV*

Never Watch	41%
12 - 2 p.m.	30%
2 - 4 p.m.	9%
4 - 6 p.m.	1%
6 - 8 p.m.	9%
8 - 10 p.m.	6%
10 - 12 p.m.	1%
Anytime & N.C.	3%

Never Watch 41%

Table B-5. Favorites: Newspapers

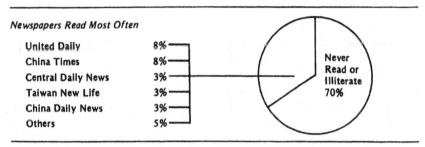

Newspapers Read Most Often	
United Daily	8%
China Times	8%
Central Daily News	3%
Taiwan New Life	3%
China Daily News	3%
Others	5%

Never Read or Illiterate 70%

Table B-6. Favorites: Magazines

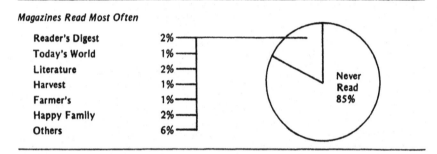

Magazines Read Most Often	
Reader's Digest	2%
Today's World	1%
Literature	2%
Harvest	1%
Farmer's	1%
Happy Family	2%
Others	6%

Never Read 85%

The best payoffs if the approach is to reach all wives twenty through forty-four would seem to be as follows:

1. buy radio time at noon to 2 p.m. when the Taiwanese Opera is on;
2. get press releases to or purchase column space at the *China Times* and *United Daily* newspapers;
3. get TV time from noon to 2 p.m., running ads while the Taiwanese Opera is on;
4. continue showing slides and films at movie theaters, but be certain that they give detailed, specific information; and
5. forget magazines unless cost is minimal: *Harvest* should be dropped (it costs US$2,500 yearly and less than 1 per cent have seen it); *Farmer's Magazine* has more readers and costs only one-tenth the price of *Harvest*.

POINT 4: SELECTING AUDIENCES TO REACH

In order of need to curb fertility, the rural and uneducated ought to be high priority. Those not practicing family planning methods ought to be a select target. *Highest* should be those who want no more children but are not practicing (the latter likely ready to practice and needing motivation). Highest priority should go to those not knowing how to use methods. Husbands ought to be considered as secondary targets as well as younger wives who may need to be motivated to practice rather than just informed about a contraceptive service. The following help identify the methods to use to reach these selected target groups:

Priority Target 1a: Rural Women

1. Use Taiwanese Opera and Taiwanese popular songs on radio as the best vehicle (25% of all rural townships wives listen most often to Taiwanese Opera and 10% to Taiwanese popular songs). The radio time to buy is from 12-2 p.m. or, as second choice, 8-12 p.m.
2. Use Taiwanese Opera on TV (since 30% of all rural wives listened most often to this format) and/or buy time from 12-2 p.m. (again 30% listed most often here).
3. Forget newspapers and magazines with this group; also keep in mind that only (or as many as) 9 per cent had ever seen family planning posters.

Priority Target 1b: Uneducated Wives

1. Use radio with Taiwanese Opera (30% of uneducated wives listed it as the one usually listened to). A poor second choice is Taiwanese popular songs or Taiwanese plays. The best time to buy by far is 12-2 p.m. (25% list it as usually listening).
2. TV may be a low-priority possibility (since 40% of the uneducated watch it sometimes but only 20% watch it as often as once or twice weekly). Only Taiwanese Opera would be worthwhile for the uneducated though (1 of 3 mention it was usually watched), and only 12-2 p.m. is prime time (1 of 3 choosing it).
3. Movies are possible but only 1 of 5 goes and less than once a month.
4. Newspapers and magazines should be forgotten. Furthermore, our *posters do not reach the uneducated* (only 3% saw them).

Priority Target 2: Wives Younger Than Thirty Years

1. *Radio* programs combining Chinese popular and Taiwanese popular songs are best choice (20% of wives twenty through twenty-nine years old list these two as usual favorites) and the best times are 12-2 p.m. and 8-12 p.m.
2. *TV* with either Taiwanese Opera or Chinese and Taiwanese popular songs combined is a good choice (13% of wives listed the songs). The best time is 12-2 p.m., a second choice is 6-8 p.m.

3. Only 7 per cent go once a month to *movies* but this is more than wives thirty or more.
4. 12 per cent of wives twenty through twenty-nine read newspapers daily and the *United Daily* and *China Times* are the big favorites.

Priority Target 3: Husbands

1. Movie theaters and newspapers are unusually good approaches to reach husbands (33% go to movies at least once monthly and 38% read newspapers daily).

POINT 5: IDENTIFYING GROUPS

Those not practicing methods and also those who are not practicing and do not want more children are groups that can be identified. A few suggestions are made without benefit of breakdown by age, area, or education.

Those Not Practicing (56% of All Wives)

1. Use radio at 12-2 p.m., either Taiwanese Opera or a show with Chinese and Taiwanese popular songs.
2. TV with Taiwanese Opera at 12-2 p.m.
3. Movies are possible (8% went once a month; 40% go but most less than once a month).
4. Newspapers are possible with the *United Daily* and *China News*.
5. 10 per cent had seen the family planning posters.

Those Not Practicing and Not Wanting More Children (23% of All Wives)

1. Radio with Taiwanese Opera 12-2 p.m. (21%) is best; Chinese and popular songs reach 13 per cent; Taiwanese plays reach 7 per cent.
2. TV is well worthwhile with 20 per cent watching daily and 50 per cent watching sometimes. Taiwanese Opera is the best bet (29%) and 12-2 p.m. (20%); 2-4 p.m. (8%) and 6-8 p.m. (6%) are second choices.
3. Newspapers are read by 19 per cent and 8 per cent daily — the *United Daily* and *China Times* are the favorites.

Content here should be informational and specific.

APPENDIX
C

MASS MAILING PROPOSALS: ICARP COUNTRIES

*A memo to the International Committee for
Applied Research on Population (ICARP) to illustrate
by Taiwan's experience, the possibilities for
the use of mailing campaigns in Asian countries.
Questions raised are answered.*

MEMORANDUM

Date: 13 April 1973

To: ICARP Members

From: George P. Cernada

Subject: Mass Mailing Proposals: ICARP Countries

At the Taipei session, several colleagues requested that a general protocol for a mass mailing project for ICARP countries be drawn up for review at the next meeting. There, however, is not enough information on each country's study objective, the audience to be reached, the kind of message to be conveyed, the quality of the listing of mailing recipients or the effectiveness of the mailing system to do so. I, therefore, have put together this instructional kit for your reference.

This kit is in four parts:

1. *Questions and Answers About Mass Mailings* (A Dialogue Between a True Believer and a Skeptic);
2. *Possible Project Proposals*;
3. *A Sample Postpartum Letter* (w/return coupon); and
4. *Summary Review of Mailing Approaches* (in India, Korea, Hong Kong, and Taiwan).

If after reviewing, you wish to draft a protocol geared to your needs, I could work individually with you during the Manila session.

QUESTIONS AND ANSWERS

Q1: *Is it true that Mass Mailings in Asia have had some success but have not been tried enough?*

> **A1:** Yes. Both India and Taiwan have tried successful mailing approaches, particularly to women recently having had a baby (Taiwan) and community leaders (India). Korea's experience has been mixed, Hong Kong's less favorable. An article describing these experiences is attached. Much more could be done!

Q2: *What are the reasons why it has not been used more extensively?*

> **A2:** Probably partly because the general use of mass approaches has been limited in some places. Some also believe that the postal systems are not very useful, that getting mailing lists are difficult, that too many people are illiterate to read, that it costs too much, that you never know if it works or not, etc.

Q3: *Which of the above criticisms of mailing seem valid?*

> **A3:** None. It is likely that there are few developing countries today where some sort of mailing approach could not be used effectively to reach an intended audience at a low cost.

Q4: *What about a country where the government is relunctant to use Mass Media?*

> **A4:** An ideal situation! Taiwan placed a good deal of attention on mailing at one stage because there was no Government policy and mailing was considered no more "mass" or "public" in approach than home-visiting and much less controversial than TV or radio or newspaper approaches.

Q5: *But what if the postal system is weak? How can you know that the letter reached the person you intended it to?*

> **A5:** Whether a letter reaches a person, of course, depends not only on the postal system or the mailman but also on the house addressing system in the area (e.g., Does a house have a number?) and also the accuracy of the mailing list you have. But if you mail 100,000 letters which cost US$2,500 for postage, printing and labor and only 80,000 letters reach their destination, is it not worth the cost — particularly if 3,000 came to a clinic for contraceptive method?

Q6: *But how do you find out whether the mail will reach people you want it to?*

A6: That should be easy. First, you randomly sample a 1,000 from the 100,000 list and mail only to them. Then after a month or so (or whatever grace period is suitable locally), you go to the post office and see how many letters were returned to you as undeliverable and why. To expedite the process, you provide a gift to the post office clerk to put these aside for you.

If the return delivery system is not used in your country, you sample 10 per cent of the 1,000 and go to them to find out whether they received the mail.

Q7: *What can you do beforehand to be sure it arrives?*

A7: The best bet is getting an accurate up-to-date mailing list. Find out if any commercial firms have one. The birth registration system can be the best of all since it is often up-to-date and you know you have a fertile woman.

Q8: *But not all babies born are registered.*

A8: Well, mail only to those who are. If 400,000 babies are born a year in your country and only a quarter are registered, then there are 100,000 you can mail to. In some countries, baptismal records may be the better source for new borns.

Q9: *But what if there is no large general audience you can reach?*

A9: Then be selective. The more selective your mailing list is the better chance for results. Try the medical association for private doctors. The religious groups for ministers. The government organizations for community leaders. The large city hospitals for the addresses of mothers recently delivering.

In some cases you may want to influence leaders; in some, recruit acceptors.

Q10: *How can you know if people will read the letter?*

A10: Find out by asking and observing. Illiterate wives may have educated husbands or children or relatives who can read to them. In some villages the headman reads the correspondence to the recipient. A follow-up survey can be conducted to find out.

Q11: *What else can you do to be sure someone reads the letter?*

A11: Make it vital, alive, interesting. Appeal to their interests: "Congratulations to you on your new baby! A special offer only for you should you decide to postpone the next child!!!" Try the "limited time only" offer to increase returns.

Most importantly, try out your message beforehand — not just with your colleagues but also with the people you will send the letters to. Pretest! Find out what the intended recipient thinks about your letter. Ask her to write it, even!

Q12: *You're beginning to convince me but won't it cost a lot? You know how the boys back home are about "cost-effectiveness"?*

A12: If that is all that is holding you back, you are ready to consult your Taiwan colleagues who will help you draft a protocol! In one Asian country the cost per mailing (including printing, postage, and labor) is only US2.5¢ per letter. Imagine — your message delivered 250 miles away up country to Dr. Rosenfield for only 2.5¢!! They had a return of 5 per cent — i.e., 5 of every 100 come in for IUD insertion or an average cost of US$2.50 per 5 cases of US50¢ each. See the list of possible project proposals attached!

Q13: *But how will you know who accepted?*

A13: Easy. Try the return coupon system Korea and Taiwan use. Adapt it to your situation. A sample is attached.

Q14: *Rather than leave the number of questions at our unlucky thirteen, let's try one last one, OK? Do you think we could get a little outside support? You know, a few (dollars, baht, yen, won, pesos) to help us devote our enthusiastic attention to this project and avoid all the usual local red tape.*

A14: See John Ross now.

POSSIBLE PROJECT PROPOSALS (PILOT TESTS)

Projects	Purpose
General	
1. *Large-scale mass mailing to recent postpartum cases*	Increased Contraceptive Acceptance
2. *Large-scale to all couples w/two or more children*	Increased Contraceptive Acceptance
3. *Large-scale to all acceptors prior to 1972*	To increase Continuation by offering Contraception (e.g., other methods to former pill users)
4. *Large-scale to all newlyweds*	Marriage Manual or Return Information Coupon
Special Groups	
5. *All private physicians*	To Encourage Cooperation, Solicit Information, Provide Materials for Distribution
6. *All school teachers*	To Inform about Program

7. *All local leaders*	To Suggest Ways to Help Program
8. *All religious leaders*	To Identify Common Goals in F. P. Service
9. *All home economists*	To Show How They Can Integrate F. P. in Their Extension or Teaching
10. *All Farmers' Association members*	To Show How They Can Integrate F. P. in Their Extension or Teaching
11. *Workers in large industries*	Offer Contraceptive Information and Services

The above are only a few of many possible projects. In some countries, all could be done; in others, an ineffective mailing system to rural areas or a weak birth registration system might make some projects more difficult to carry out. Program priorities also differ from place to place.

Some might wish to carry out a general mass mailing (e.g., projects numbers 1 through 4 above) while others would focus on a special group whose addresses might be available more easily (e.g., numbers 5 through 11).

Others less certain of results might wish to first study one or more of the following:

1. whether the mail reaches the intended audience;
2. whether it is read;
3. which kind of message gets better results (Taiwan has tried this);
4. whether mailing lists can be composed(e.g., would baptismal records in the Philippines be a better source of postpartum cases than municipality registration offices?);
5. whether a simple return coupon system can be used for easier evaluation; and
6. whether a mailing system could be integrated into an ongoing service (e.g., postpartum maternity hospital referral service to sector health centers in Bangkok).*

---

* EDITOR'S NOTE: Sample Postpartum Letter and Summary Review of Mailing Approaches not included here. For a review of mailing trials in various countries, see Cernada [34].

APPENDIX
D

BIRTH SPACING INCENTIVE PLAN: TAICHUNG

Description of innovative project to provide incentives to couples to space between children for three-year periods. Pilot project was implemented in Taiwan in 1975.

GRANT REQUEST TO INTERNATIONAL COMMITTEE FOR APPLIED RESEARCH ON POPULATION

Summary Sheet

1. *Lead:* Incentive Scheme for Postponing Births

2. *Amount:* US$34,000

    XX   : a. Pay entire amount at once.

    ————— : b. Pay in four quarterly installments, the first one at once.

    ————— : c. Other – Specify: _____

3. *Grant Period:* From *1/Apr/73* to *31/Mar/77* (when final report is done)

4. *Grantee:* Institution: *National Health Administration and Joint Commission on Rural Reconstruction (JCRR)*
               Address: *37, Nanhai Road, Taipei, Republic of China*
               Principal Investigator: *Dr. C. M. Wang*
                           c/o Committee on Family Planning
                           P.O. Box 1020, Taichung, Taiwan
               Send Payments to: *JCRR, 37 Nanhai Road, Taipei, ROC*

5. *Title of Project:* *PLANNED FAMILY PILOT PROJECT*

6. *Purpose:* (1) To determine if married couples ages fifteen to twenty-nine in Taichung City with only one child can be persuaded to enroll in a program designed to provide educational and contraceptive services in order to postpone birth of a second child for a minimum of three years spacing. The incentive will be free delivery and hospital care for those who succeed and nutritional supplements for children.

(2) For the Taiwan Provincial Health Department to present the findings at the end of three years to the Taiwan Provincial Government to persuade them to provide these free medical services to all couples who space children accordingly. It is hoped that this project also will increase the safety of deliveries and strengthen the present postpartum program at the Provincial Hospitals.

(3) To provide a baseline of knowledge about this incentive approach and its success in order to better plan for future implementation of a more comprehensive program providing incentives for postponing marriage, first birth (as well as second), and stopping at two children.

7. *Budget:* The cost is US$34,000: US$24,000 for costs of deliveries and related hospital care and nutritional supplements and $10,000 for administrative costs. Staffing and evaluation will be provided through the Taiwan Provincial Health Department's Committee on Family Planning as will the free contraceptive services. The Government program investment: $10,000 — for staffing and related costs.

Research Plan

1. *Objectives:*

a. To carry out an action plan in Taichung City (capital city of the Province of Taiwan) to enroll all couples, after the birth of their first child, in an educational and incentive-oriented program to promote expanding the mean open birth interval from the *present mean of 23.7 months to 36, 42, or 48 months and beyond.*

b. To reward all those who enroll by providing free contraceptive and additional educational services. For those who reach three years without a birth free delivery service for their second child (as well as hospital care and other services for those who continue longer without a second child) will be provided.

c. For the Taiwan Provincial Health Department to demonstrate to the Taiwan Provincial Government that this service is:
   (i) worth providing on a larger scale due to its maternal health and demographic values; and
   (ii) easily replicable by having public Provincial and County Hospitals (now under the authority of the Provincial Health Department and Taiwan Provincial Government) provide this free delivery and maternity care.

d. To expand the project at the end of two years to include similar incentives:
   (i) for postponing marriage;
   (ii) for postponing a first child for a minimum of two years; and
   (iii) for continuing periods of non-fertility after the second child.

2. Background:

Taiwan has carried out successfully a variety of incentive projects in the past eight years of active family planning programming. In 1971 it even initiated its first non-fertility incentive scheme and after a year, 98 per cent of initial enrollees have re-enrolled. It is believed that economic planners are interested enough to carry out an incentive scheme which can be easily incorporated into the present government service capacity. This present project involves providing free care largely at the Taichung Provincial Hospital, which, if successful, could be expanded to all other urban areas (which have similar hospital facilities). The project itself could serve also as a point of expansion for similar incentive-oriented appeals to women with no children or those who ought to remain at two – particularly now that the new Governor of Taiwan Province has indicated the importance of the two-child ideal and the national Minister of Finance has publicly expressed the need for families to consider two children as the ideal.

It is hoped that this project will bring the present mean interval between the first and second child from 23.7 to about 42 months or almost double the time length for 1971.

3. Plan of Action:

a. Procedure

Extensive pre-publicity will be carried out. Small bonuses to district legislation offices, health stations, and other city agency leaders will be provided for meeting local recruitment targets. The Taichung City Government will be involved actively in project implementation. Staff will be provided by the Taiwan Committee on Family Planning, the Maternal and Child Health Institute (both headquartered in Taichung), and the Taichung City Health Bureau. Those who enroll will be provided contraceptive services (pill, loop, condom) at no charge. They also will be provided educational services, counseling, and be exposed to a local radio series on the subject of spacing. Each enrolling couple will receive a card indicating the date of enrollment and a leaflet describing the bonuses they are eligible for and when. Our previous recruiting experience with the educational savings plan, sponsored by the Population Council, will be helpful here.

b. *Enrollment*

It is estimated that 3,100 women fifteen to twenty-nine will have a first birth during the first year of the project (based on 1972 data — See Tables following). It is hoped to recruit a minimum of 90 per cent of these. Of those 2,800 enrolling, we estimate that the mean open interval between first and second births can be raised from the present estimated 23.7 months to approximately 40 months. The distribution of second births over the four years would be as follows:

Status	Number of Wives	Estimated Mean Open Birth Interval
1. Not Enrolling	300	24 Months
2. Enrolling But Having Second Child Before 36 Months Interval	500	27 Months
3. Enrolling and Not Having Second Child Before 36 Months Interval	1,000	40 Months
4. Enrolling and Not Having Second Child Before 42 Months Interval	700	46 Months
5. Enrolling and Not Having Second Child Before 48 Months Interval	600	52 Months
Total	3,100	With Mean Open Birth Interval of 40 Months

c. *Education*

Names of mothers having babies are now copied from local registration offices for our postpartum approach. Those who have had first births will be visited by a specially-trained family planning field worker to explain the program and enroll the new mother within two months of her first baby's birth. Women enrolling will attend special "mother's classes" focusing on health and economic reasons for postponing a second child and also receive special postnatal mother and child care lessons. These sessions will be held regularly. A special radio program will be arranged to supplement the group meetings as well as educational materials prepared.

d. *Bonuses* (US$24,000-approximately)

The bonuses for those postponing births will be as follows.

	Step 1 (36 Mos.)	Step 2 (42 Mos.)	Step 3 (48 Mos.)
Postponing Second Child:	Free delivery (US$5.00) of second child at Taichung Prov. Hospital or equivalent payment to private doctor, midwife plus related expenses (US$2.50).	Same as Step 1 plus free hospital care expenses for mother and child.	Same as Step 2 plus powdered milk, food supplements for infant during first year.
	1,000 couples @ Avg. US$7.50 each = *$7,500*	700 cases @ Avg. US$10 each = *$7,000*	600 couples @ Avg. US$15 each = *$9,000*

In order not to encourage the second child, it will be made clear to all participants that they can receive the bonus in cash (in lieu of services) at 36 months or thereafter according to the payments specified above.

e. *Future Possible Incentive Plans*

If this plan meets with some success, those couples enrolled in it would be eligible for a second plan (which would be the subject of a separate request for funding). The next plan would be to provide incentives related to kindergarten and related child care costs for those who do not have second or third children. In addition, a similar plan focusing in the same way on postponing the first child mean open interval of fifteen months would be implemented (to extend it to two years, thirty months, and three years periods) if funding is made available. The three plans would cover the entire childbearing period. Estimated costs of Plan A (postponing child 1) would be US$15,000; of Plan C (stopping at two), approximate funds US$50,000; Plan B (described in this request) costs US$24,000 in incentive bonus.

f. *Administration/Evaluation*

US$10,000 total. Matching services of approximately US$10,000 in supporting staff costs to be provided by the Taiwan Provincial Health Department.

The US$10,000 will be used to cover costs of the educational campaign (travel money, radio time, educational materials, group meetings) and for the concise inventory of records that will be necessary to evaluate the progress of the program.

Evaluation

Evaluation will consist of:

1. *Immediate*
   a. Per cent of eligibles able to be reached and enrolled. 90 per cent is the goal. A continuing series of service statistics on characteristics of acceptors vs. non-acceptors will be maintained. Non-enrollees will be visited after a period to find out why they have not enrolled.

2. *Intermediate*
   b. Per cent of attendance at "mother's classes" will be maintained. Observation of interest of mothers at educational sessions will be carried out. A pre- and post-attendance survey will be carried out in regard to knowledge, attitude and contraceptive practice.
   c. A review of birth registers will be carried out monthly after the first nine months in order to determine whether women enrolled have become pregnant and to observe the general birth rate trend in the age group.
   d. Records of all contraceptive acceptors through the general family planning program will be reviewed on a quarterly basis to find out if those in the plan are accepting contraceptive methods.

3. *Longer-Term*
   e. The mean birth interval, standard deviation, and time distribution of open birth intervals (for mothers fifteen through twenty-nine) for the year 1972 (in Taichung City) will be calculated.[1] These figures will be matched with the results of the special program to be carried out over 1973, 1974, and 1975. Breakdowns by age groups, education and related variables will be carried out.
   f. Those enrolled in the program also will be compared with non-enrollees for length of open birth intervals.
   g. A control city, Tainan, has been selected to determine what progress in lengthening open birth interval would have taken place anyway (i.e., without our special incentive program). For comparative details, see Tables following.
   h. A follow-up interview of a sample of successful and unsuccessful enrollees will be carried out after a review of the characteristics associated with successful participation.

---

[1] NOTE: Our present mean interval and distribution of 23.7 months is based upon the Taichung City sample from the 1970 KAP III survey — see Tables. We propose to review the actual records of the 3,000 births in Taichung (1972) after the project begins.

Table D-1. Numbers of First Live Births by Mother's Age
(15-29): 1972 (Taichung City)

Age	Number of Live Births
15 - 19	355
20 - 24	2,843
25 - 29	768
Total	2,966

SOURCE: Birth registration data at Taichung City
district registration offices. Compiled
initially for family planning program's postpartum mailing and home-visiting approach
by health station family planning workers.

Table D-2. Percentage Distribution of Wives by Open Length of
Second Live Birth Intervals: Taichung City (Experimental Area)
(from KAP III Survey, 1970)[a]

Age	Number of Wives	No Births	Per Cent Wives in Each Interval					
			0-6	6-12	12-18	18-24	24-30	30+
22-29	64	37.5	0	4.7	10.9	20.3	15.6	10.9
30-42	107	0.9	0	0	19.6	32.7	20.6	26.2
22-42	171	14.6	0	1.8	16.4	28.1	18.7	20.5

Mean Length of Open Interval: 23.7 Months (Ages 22-29)
27.4 Months (Ages 30-42)
26.4 Months (Ages 22-42)

[a] This computation is based upon the 171 Taichung City wives who had a first live birth
in the Island-wide KAP survey (1970). The actual intervals and distributions for 1972 and
on for Taichung City will be gathered from the vital data at the registration offices after
receipt of funds for the project.

Table D-3. Percentage Distribution of Wives by Open Length of
Second Live Birth Intervals: Tainan City (Control Area)
(from KAP III Survey, 1970)[a]

Age	No. of Wives	Per Cent Wives in Each Interval						
		No Births	0-6	6-12	12-18	18-24	24-30	30+
22-29	53	22.6	0	1.9	18.9	26.4	17.0	13.2
30-42	72	1.4	1.4	2.8	18.1	31.9	22.2	22.2
22-42	125	10.4	0.8	2.4	18.4	29.6	20.0	18.4

Mean Length of Second Live Birth Interval is: 24.5 Months (Ages 22-29)
25.8 Months (Ages 30-42)
25.3 Mohths (Ages 22-42)

[a] Actual vital data will be gathered at Tainan registration offices for 1972 and on.

Table D-4. Number of Women Marrying in Taichung and Tainan Cities in 1972

City	Age at Marriage		
	Below 30	Above 30	Total
Taichung	2,818	955	3,773
Tainan	2,940	789	3,729

Table D-5. Estimated Per Cent of Wives (Ages 20-29) Who Had One
Child in Taichung and Tainan Cities by Age of Wife (1971)[a]

Age	Number of Wives		Per Cent With One Child: Both Cities
	Taichung	Tainan	
15-19	1,281	1,332	42.1
20-24	9,394	9,429	33.2
25-29	13,296	13,216	14.5

[a] Based on "percentage distribution by parity of ever-married women by age by family
type for eight urban townships in Taiwan" (Table 7-3), Demographic Monthly, Republic of
China, July 1971.

Table D-6. Population Age Distribution by Sex, End of 1971:
Taichung and Tainan Cities as Matching Experimental/Control Areas

	Taichung City	Tainan City
Male	242,950	252,146
Female	224,367	232,553
Total	467,317	484,699

Table D-7. Female Population Distribution by Ages 15-29, End of 1971:
Taichung and Tainan Cities as Matching Experimental/Control Areas)

Ages	Taichung City	Tainan City
15-19	26,092	27,476
20-24	22,303	23,396
25-29	15,871	15,817
Total	64,266	66,689

Table D-8. Numbers of Births and Marriages During 1971:
Taichung and Tainan Cities as Matching Experimental/Control Areas

Event	Taichung City	Tainan City
Births	11,260	11,909
Marriages	3,413	3,437

Table D-9. Crude Birth, Death, Natural Increase Rates, 1971:
Taichung and Tainan Cities as Matching Experimental/Control Areas

	Taichung City	Tainan City
Crude Birth Rate	24.60	24.82
Crude Death Rate	4.05	4.39
Natural Increase Rate	20.55	20.43

Table D-10. Cumulative Numbers of Contraceptive Acceptors
(Program-Supplied) and Rate of Contraceptive
Acceptances Among Wives 20-44 (End 1971):
Taichung and Tainan Cities as Matching Experimental/Control Areas

Method	Taichung City		Tainan City	
	Number	Per Cent[a]	Number	Per Cent[a]
Loop	30,053	52.8	33,041	55.5
Pill	8,918	15.7	10,245	17.2
Condom	5,853	10.3	3,742	6.3

[a] Rate of acceptance (including reinsertion of loop) among total
wives 20-44, end 1970 (56,908 in Taichung; 59,574 in Tainan).

REFERENCES

1. B. Berelson, The World Population Plan of Action: Where Now?, *Population and Development Review*, 2:2, pp. 219-266, 1976.
2. J. Echols (ed.), *Making Population-Family Planning Research Useful: The Communicator's Contribution*, Conference Summary Report, East-West Communication Institute, Honolulu, Hawaii, April 1974.
3. E. H. Spicer, *Human Problems in Technological Change: A Casebook*, Wiley and Sons, New York, 1967.
4. B. D. Paul, *Health, Culture and Community*, Russell Sage, New York, 1961.
5. R. G. Havelock, *Planning for Innovation: Through Dissemination and Utilization of Knowledge*, Center for Research on Utilization of Scientific Knowledge, Institute for Social Research, University of Michigan, Ann Arbor, 1971.
6. E. M. Rogers, *Communication Strategies for Family Planning*, The Free Press, New York, 1973.
7. G. P. Cernada and T. H. Sun, Knowledge Into Action: The Use of Research in Taiwan's Family Planning Program, *East-West Communication Institute Papers Series*, East-West Center, Honolulu, No. 10, 1976.
8. R. Reynolds, S. J. Haider, and N. I. Khan, Process, Content, Action — Training Family Planning Workers as Agents of Social Change, *International Journal of Health Education*, 16:2, pp. 126-135, 1973.
9. A. Knutson, Evaluation for What?, H. C. Shulberg, A. Sheldon and F. Baker (eds.), *Program Evaluation in the Health Fields*, Behavioral Publications, New York, 1969.

10. N. I. Khan and R. Reynolds, Strategies for Achieving Research Utilization in the Bangladesh Population Program: Implications for Health Education, *International Quarterly of Community Health Education, 1:2*, pp. 135-152, 1981.

11. S. B. Kar, Management and Utilization of Population Communication Research, *A Synthesis of Population Communication Experience*, Paper 5, East-West Communication Institute, Honolulu, Hawaii, July 1977.

12. B. Roberts, Scientific Group: Research in Health Education, *Background Paper*, World Health Organization, Geneva, p. 1, December 1968.

13. Human Interaction Research Institute, *Putting Knowledge to Use: A Distillation of the Literature Regarding Knowledge Transfer and Change*, Los Angeles, pp. 5-8, 1976.

14. L. W. Green, et al., *Health Education Planning: A Diagnostic Approach*, Mayfield Publishing, Palo Alto, California, p. 127, 1980.

15. Rogers, pp. 394-396, 1973.

16. R. K. Merton, L. Brown, and L. S. Cottrell, *Sociology Today*, Basic Books, New York, p. 21, 1959.

17. P. H. Tannenbaum, Communication of Science Information, *Science, 140*, p. 580, May 10, 1963.

18. B. E. Grey, Information and Research — Blood Relatives or In-Laws? Dissemination of the Results of Experimentation is an Integral Part of the Total Research Process, *Science, 137*, pp. 263-266, July 1962.

19. S. M. Keeny, G. P. Cernada, T. C. Hsu, T. H. Sun, S. C. Hsu, and L. P. Chow, Taiwan, *Country Profile Series*, The Population Council, New York, February 1970.

20. E. C. Cernada and G. P. Cernada, Taiwan, W. Watson (ed.), *Family Planning in the Developing World*, The Population Council, New York, pp. 22-24, 1977.

21. C. M. Wang and T. H. Sun, Taiwan, *Studies in Family Planning, 9:9*, pp. 247-250, 1978.

22. J. R. Echols, 1974.

23. N. I. Khan and R. Reynolds, 1981.

24. S. B. Kar, 1977.

25. S. M. Keeny, et al., February 1970.

26. E. C. Cernada and G. P. Cernada, 1977.

27. G. P. Cernada and T. H. Sun, 1976.

28. C. M. Wang and T. H. Sun, 1978.

29. R. Freedman, L. C. Coombs, M. C. Chang, and T. H. Sun, Trends in Fertility, Family Size Preferences, and Practice of Family Planning, Taiwan, 1965-1973, *Studies in Family Planning, 5*, pp. 269-288, 1974.

30. R. Cuca and C. S. Pierce, *Experiments in Family Planning: Lessons From the Developing World*, World Bank, Washington, D.C., 1977.

31. B. Berelson and R. Freedman, A Study in Fertility Control, *Scientific American, 210:5*, pp. 3-11, 1964.

32. M. C. Chang, G. P. Cernada, and T. H. Sun, A Fieldworker Incentive Experimental Study, *Studies in Family Planning, 3:*11, pp. 270-272, 1972.
33. G. P. Cernada and L. P. Lu, The Kaohsiung Study, *Studies in Family Planning, 3:*8, pp. 198-203, 1972.
34. G. P. Cernada, Direct Mailings to Promote Family Planning, *Studies in Family Planning, 1:*53, pp. 16-19, 1970.
35. J. Ross, et al., Findings From Family Planning Research, *Reports on Population/Family Planning, 12,* Population Council, New York, 1972.
36. R. Gillespie, L. P. Chow, and H. C. Chen, Taiwan: Experimental Series, *Studies in Family Planning, 1:*13, pp. 1-5, 1966.
37. O. D. Finnigan and T. H. Sun, Planning, Starting, and Operating an Educational Incentive Project, *Studies in Family Planning, 3:*1, pp. 1-7, 1972.
38. G. P. Cernada and L. P. Chow, The Coupon System in an Ongoing Family Planning Program, *American Journal of Public Health, 59:*12, pp. 2199-2208, 1969.
39. R. Freedman and J. Y. Takeshita, *Family Planning in Taiwan: An Experiment in Social Change,* Princeton University Press, New Jersey, 1969.
40. G. P. Cernada, *Taiwan Family Planning Reader: How a Program Works,* Chinese Center for International Training in Family Planning, P. O. Box 112, Taichung, Taiwan, 1970.
41. Chinese Center for International Training in Family Planning, *Annotated Taiwan Population Bibliography,* Taichung, Taiwan, 1974.
42. Taiwan Committee on Family Planning, *Taiwan Population Studies Summaries,* Taichung, Taiwan, 1973.
43. Chinese Center for International Training in Family Planning, *Family Planning Communications in Taiwan Area, Republic of China,* 2nd edition, Taichung, Taiwan, 1973.
44. E. A. Golda, A Philatelic View, *Family Planning Perspectives, 4,* pp. 7-8, 1972.
45. Chinese Center for International Training in Family Planning, *Paste Your Umbrella Before The Rain,* Taichung, Taiwan, p. 3, 1973.
46. *Ibid.,* pp. 3-4.
47. Cuca and Pierce, p. 3.
48. Cernada and Sun, p. 15.
49. Finnigan and Sun, pp. 1-7.
50. C. M. Wang and S. Y. Chen, Evaluation of the First Year of the Educational Savings Program in Taiwan, *Studies in Family Planning, 4:*7, pp. 157-161, 1973.
51. Cernada and Sun, p. 18.
52. *Taiwan's Health: 1963,* Taichung, Taiwan, 1964.
53. D. Nyswander, Education for Health: Some Principles and Their Application, *Health Education Conference,* Chapel Hill, North Carolina, March 21, 1956.

54. K. Lewin, *Field Theory in Social Science*, Harper, New York, 1951.
55. H. Lasswell and A. Kaplan, *Power and Society: A Framework for Political Inquiry*, Yale, 1950.
56. B. Berelson, Communication and Public Opinion, W. Schramm (ed.), *The Process and Effects of Mass Communication*, University of Illinois, Urbana, pp. 342-356, 1961.
57. G. Cernada, Population Policy, Programs and Social and Economic Development Planning in Developing Countries, International Congress of World Federation of Public Health Associations, Halifax, Nova Scotia, Canada, 1978.
58. P. Mullen and R. Reynolds, The Potential of Grounded Theory for Health Education Research: Linking Theory and Practice, *Health Education Monographs*, 5:3, pp. 280-294, 1978.
59. G. Watson, *Concepts for Social Change*, Cooperative Project for Educational Development, NTL Institute for Applied Behavioral Science, Washington, D.C., 1976.
60. R. Lippitt, J. Watson, and B. Westley, *The Dynamics of Planned Change*, Harcourt, Brace, New York, 1958.
61. R. Miles, Human Relations or Human Resources?, *Harvard Business Review*, 43:4, pp. 148-156, 1965.
62. C. Jung and R. Lippitt, *Utilization of Scientific Knowledge for Change in Education*, CRUSK, University of Michigan, Ann Arbor, 1969.
63. G. Allport, Perception and Public Health, *Health Education Monographs*, No. 2, 1958.
64. M. B. Smith, A Social-Psychological View of Fertility, J. Fawcett (ed.), *Psychological Perspectives on Population*, Basic Books, New York, pp. 3-18, 1973.
65. W. Wohlking, Attitude Change, Behavior Change, *California Management Review*, 13:2, pp. 45-50, 1970.
66. W. Goodenough, *Cooperation in Change*, Russell Sage, New York, p. 42, 1963.
67. J. Nyerere, *Education for Self-Reliance*, Government Printer, Dar Es Salaam, United Republic of Tanzania, March 1967.
68. P. Friere, *Pedagogy For The Oppressed*, Penquin, England, 1972.
69. G. Pine and P. Horn, Principles of Learning, *Adult Leadership*, pp. 108-110, October 1969.